High Stakes

HIGH STAKES
THE CRITICAL ROLE OF STAKEHOLDERS IN HEALTH CARE

David A. Shore
with
Eric D. Kupferberg

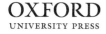

Oxford University Press, Inc., publishes works that further
Oxford University's objective of excellence
in research, scholarship, and education.

Oxford   New York
Auckland   Cape Town   Dar es Salaam   Hong Kong   Karachi
Kuala Lumpur   Madrid   Melbourne   Mexico City   Nairobi
New Delhi   Shanghai   Taipei   Toronto

With offices in
Argentina   Austria   Brazil   Chile   Czech Republic   France   Greece
Guatemala   Hungary   Italy   Japan   Poland   Portugal   Singapore
South Korea   Switzerland   Thailand   Turkey   Ukraine   Vietnam

Copyright © 2011 by David A. Shore.

Published by Oxford University Press, Inc.
198 Madison Avenue, New York, New York 10016
www.oup.com

Oxford is a registered trademark of Oxford University Press

All rights reserved. No part of this publication may be reproduced,
stored in a retrieval system, or transmitted, in any form or by any means,
electronic, mechanical, photocopying, recording, or otherwise,
without the prior permission of Oxford University Press.

Library of Congress Cataloging-in-Publication Data

Shore, David A., 1954- author.
High stakes : the critical role of stakeholders in
health care / David A. Shore ; with Eric D. Kupferberg.
p. ; cm.
Includes bibliographical references.
ISBN 978-0-19-532625-3
1. Medical policy—United States. 2. Medical care—United States.
I. Kupferberg, Eric D., author. II. Title.
  [DNLM: 1. Health Care Sector—organization & administration—United States.
2. Economic Competition—United States. 3. Health Services Needs and
Demand—United States. 4. Interpersonal Relations—United States.
5. Negotiating—United States. W 74 AA1]
RA395.A3S494 2011
362.10973—dc22
2010045919

Printed in the United States of America
on acid-free paper
9 8 7 6 5 4 3 2 1

To the stakeholders in my life: my parents, Ruth and Milton Shore; my wife, Charlotte Shore; and my children, Douglas and Alyssa. I am a very lucky man to have you all.
—David A. Shore

For Susan Shelkrot, Leo Kupferberg, and Harvey J. Kupferberg
—Eric D. Kupferberg

Preface: Purposes, Analytical Approach, and Source Material

This book is not a diatribe. It is about a dialogue. Actually, it is the product of several dialogues: a dialogue between my collaborator and myself, a dialogue with my students, a dialogue with the participants of our executive education programs, a dialogue with my colleagues at Harvard University and other academic institutions, and a dialogue with leaders of health care institutions. These dialogues are far from finished. Part of the nature of productive dialogues is that they are ongoing. This book makes no pretence of being the final word on health care considerations. The health care landscape is in a constant state of flux. In fact, we fully anticipate that the debates and questions will shift between the time of this writing and the time that the book is published.

Nonetheless, we have written this book with the intention of its being relevant throughout the present and upcoming periods of change. As most readers will fully appreciate, the challenges and issues facing stakeholder groups in health care are long-lived. Consequently, this is not a book about health care policy. We do not endorse any reforms that fit neatly into liberal or conservative political agendas. Instead, we believe that our discussion of stakeholder groups and their interrelationships will aid in the articulation and implementation of new policies across the ideological spectrum. Our descriptions of stakeholder conflicts and our prescriptions for their remedy, we hope, will cut through and across oppositional positions. They will encourage dialogue where previously there had been either striking silence or deafening dismissal.

We expect that this book will be controversial. In fact, its relevance will ensure that it will find both favor and opposition from many key participants in health care. We welcome any heated discussion that may follow as a result of our descriptions and prescriptions. Arguments, so long as they are well focused and well intentioned, are essential tools for constructing workable solutions.

Our analysis draws from many sources. Initially, we appropriate a stakeholder model and analytical frame. The premise of this book is that the warring stakeholder parties in health care can be identified by their stated affiliations, their declared interests, and their behaviors. They are also defined by the alliances that they form and by the groups they oppose. In no other arena are there as many stakeholder groups as there are in health care. Whether they are fully understood or not, stakeholder groups define the battle lines and determine who "wins" and who "loses" in ongoing struggles. If this book offers new and unique insights into the current state of affairs, it is our use of stakeholder theory that most helped us arrive at these insights.

We are also convinced that stakeholder analysis can help health care leaders understand the forces that get in the way of forming productive relationships with other leaders and organizations. Stakeholder groups often speak past each other or do not speak at all. By understanding the relationships among neighboring stakeholder groups, health care leaders can identify untapped sources of alignment and engagement. However, we want to caution that our discussion is not harnessed to any single methodology or theory. We consider stakeholder theory to be one among many useful analytic tools—one that we have adjusted to better examine the contentious world of health care. As a later chapter will explain, we believe that stakeholder theory is "good to think with."

Our narrative makes an uncommon use of the first-person pronoun. You will find that at times the first-person singular "I" directs narrative sections, while the plural pronoun "we" drives the analytic portions. The divided use is intentional. When referring to conversations with health care leaders, academic colleagues, students, or executive education participants, the narrative reflects the dialogues that "I" have had with these persons. As for our research and analytic findings, it is a product of the nearly endless hours that "we" have spent discussing the causes and possible remedies to the current health care crisis.

My collaborator and I both work on the Forces of Change program at the Harvard School of Public Health. I founded this program nearly a decade ago with the mission of translating "theory into practice." As such, the objective of this book is to keep one foot in the library and one foot in the street (or board room, government agency, hospital, physician practice, etc.). By basing our descriptions and prescriptions on our discussions with representatives from multiple professional worlds—both academic and nonacademic—we have improved our ability to keep that divided perspective and divided audience present throughout the book.

No project is ever successfully completed without the alignment and engagement of multiple constituencies. Therefore, I end this preface with the most difficult section, the acknowledgments. As one might expect from a book on stakeholders, there are far too many contributors to single each out. I am indebted to the countless students and health care executives whom I have had the honor of teaching over the years at the "Forces of Change: New Strategies for the Evolving Health Care Marketplace" courses at the Harvard School of Public Health and the Harvard Extension School. I am equally indebted to the numerous health care leaders throughout the world whom I have had the opportunity to collaborate with and learn from over many years. More specifically, in terms of the work on this book, I wish to thank my long-term colleagues at the Harvard School of Public Health, Holly Zellweger and Christina Thompson Lively. Both have made substantial contributions to my thinking and to this book. Christina's work on the graphics and

Holly's overall management of this project were superior. I am also indebted to Julio Frenk, dean of the Harvard School of Public Health, for his remarkable vision and ongoing support. I also wish to thank Katherine Schlatter for all her fine efforts. I have had the good fortune of a fine team from Oxford University Press, led by Maura Roessner, Senior Editor; Susan Lee, Senior Production Editor; and Nicholas Liu, Assistant Editor. Finally, and most notably, I wish to thank my collaborator on this book, Dr. Eric Kupferberg. Eric and I have worked and taught together for more than a decade, and I never fail to be amazed by just how smart and analytical he is. I am so pleased that he elected to join me in preparing this manuscript. It has been a delightful and rewarding collaboration.

David A. Shore
Boston, Massachusetts
September 2010

Contents

3	**1. If We're So Good, Why Aren't We Better?**
3	1.1 The Case for Cooperators
6	1.2 The Bickering Family
8	1.3 Our Perspective on Stakeholder Theory
10	1.4 The Birth and Evolution of Stakeholder Theory
12	1.5 How Have We Evolved Systems for Cooperation among Stakeholders?
13	1.6 The No-Look Pass
17	**2. The Gordian Knot**
17	2.1 What We Get for the Dollars We Spend Here in the United States
22	2.2 What Are the Major Cost-Inflators?
28	2.3 Better, Newer, and More Promising Technology: Are All the Advances Advantages?
31	2.4 How Increasing Health Care Costs Is a Cause of Conflict
32	2.5 The Gordian Knot and the Push–Pull Dynamics of Health Care Costs
39	**3. Our Great Expectations**
39	3.1 The Viagra Effect: Societal Expectations about Good Health
42	3.2 The Flip Side to the Viagra Effect: Diminishing Health Care Access and Expectations
48	3.3 Wellness as a Moving Target: Reading the Expectations of the Many Stakeholders
52	3.4 Stakeholder Alignment and the Creation of Value
57	**4. Stakeholders in Health Care: A Field Guide to Identification and Evaluation**
57	4.1 Defining Stakeholders: Who Are They? Who Are You? Who Are We?
58	4.2 Understanding the Limitations in Defining Stakeholder Groups
62	4.3 Stakeholder Salience in the Health Care World
66	4.4 The Silos that Surround Us
69	4.5 Managing for Stakeholders in Health Care
74	**5. Desperately Seeking Stakeholder Alignment: A Case Vignette**
74	5.1 Going to War versus Seeking Alignment

76	5.2 Learning about Value through the Elimination of Waste
78	5.3 The War Veteran
80	5.4 "Clout" versus "Market Presence"
84	5.5 Revisiting Saliency Modeling

88	**6. A New Framework for Studying Stakeholder Alignment**
88	6.1 On the Subject of Appropriateness
95	6.2 The Meeting
100	6.3 A "Stress Test" for Recognizing Potential Alignment
105	6.4 Stakeholder Theory in the Context of Lean Enterprise Thinking

113	**7. Working toward Better Health and Greater Satisfaction**
113	7.1 Searching for Cost Savings
115	7.2 The Next Wave of Health Care Purchaser Cost Management
120	7.3 Case Vignette: Cisco's Value Proposition—Evaluating the Regional, National, and Global Implications
123	7.4 How Can We Identify the Value Creation Process in Health Care?

126	**8. Fry or Jump: Health Care Stakeholders and the Triggers for Change**
126	8.1 Standing on a Burning Platform
127	8.2 Putting Stakeholder Theory into Perspective
131	8.3 The Enablers: Finding Those that Can Facilitate Alignment
133	8.4 The Current Forces of Change: Better Tools and Better Utilization of These Tools
137	8.5 The Commons and Health Care in a Contemporary Context

141	Index

High Stakes

1 If We're So Good, Why Aren't We Better?

1.1 THE CASE FOR COOPERATORS

Thousands of years ago, when we lived mostly in small, hunter-gatherer communities, cooperation was the foremost way of survival, if not the key to group living. Today, we tend to take cooperation for granted. Instead we focus on our competitors and how to beat them—yet there is enormous potential in finding cooperators. Successful companies make sure they are increasing market share by gaining customers or persuading customers to leave their competitors, but these successful firms also may see potential for sharing customers. There are a great deal of examples of well-known brands that have devised ways in which to cooperate. One famous case study demonstrates how Starbucks coffee reached new consumers on United Airlines flights when the coffee became the airline's official brand in 1996. While Starbucks gained exposure to new customers less familiar with the expanding gourmet coffee brand, United Airlines benefited by being able to boast that its passengers were served only top-quality brews (Keller, 2008). Fifteen years later, there are barely any airports within the United States that don't contain one or more Starbucks coffee shops doing a swift business.

Some see this example as describing a type of cross-marketing, but what we are getting at is more evolved than simply marketing. It is a form of co-competing—competing together to enhance a brand or increase market share while using a serendipitously positioned resource. We like to use the term *co-opetition*, a composite term made popular by Ray Noorda, a pioneer of early computer networking systems (Fisher, 1992).

A more contemporary example of cooperation, or co-opetition, on a mass scale has resulted from the clever engineering and marketing of the iPhone and other Apple devices. Apple's mobile phone, the iPhone, and other Apple personal devices allow thousands of independent software developers to write, give away, and sell applications for instant use via download. The myriad applications ("apps")—some useful, others enjoyable timewasters—greatly enhance the popularity and value of Apple's blockbuster products (Boudreau & Lakhani, 2009). The independent application developers may be motivated by a spectrum of potential benefits, both financial and nonfinancial. Some may actually profit from application sales or sales from other software, while others may seek to gain recognition, promote a brand, or garner consumer information from their users (Boudreau & Lakhani, 2009). This arrangement allows both Apple and the independent developers a chance to benefit together.

We might assume that players in the world of health care are willing to cooperate because what is often at stake is the health of the patient and, on a larger scale, better health outcomes for the populations they serve. However, this is not always the case. Wanting better health outcomes, for the most part, aligns with the patient's typical goal of getting better or, if that is not possible, of simply feeling better. Individually, a physician, an insurer, a hospital, and a drug company might want better outcomes as well as better profit margins, but the latter does not exactly resonate with patients, employers, and government agencies who are the purchasers of health care. So if we ask what the stakes in health care are, the one stake that all the players can agree upon without any dispute is better health outcomes. This does not mean that we can ignore the other stakes in the health care world—and each stakeholder attaches different importance to these other stakes, as disparate as they may be.

Among those selling treatments or doing the treating in health care, we frequently hear the terms "vendor" and "supplier." Everyone refers to everyone else as a vendor. Physicians refer to pharmaceutical companies as vendors, and health insurance companies refer to physicians as suppliers. So we see different parties in health care regarded either as vendors or suppliers, but not as stakeholders. This is because interactions among groups are seen as transactions. We will argue that this sort of attitude is really counterproductive to creating the level of engagement that is required for the stakeholder alignment and the creation of value.

Really, what we need to see is a movement of stakeholders engaging one another early and often, and thinking of one another as partners in an enterprise, not just as suppliers and purchasers. Parenthetically, this is precisely what Starbucks did with the selling of coffee on United Airlines. The coffee maker did not just say, "Hey, here is our coffee; let's see what you can sell on your planes, and send us our check, please!" They actually acculturated United Airlines into the Starbucks way. They came up with ways to ensure that the quality of their coffee would not be compromised by the less-than-ideal standard brewing equipment, or by the airline's preparation and presentation of their product (Keller, 2008). Once onboard brewing upgrades were installed, United Airlines flight attendants were trained on how to prepare the Starbucks coffee. Some might characterize it as training the flight attendants to double as flying baristas.

The challenge for health care stakeholders is that many entities have multiple purposes and goals. A provider might find that it has a split purpose. For example, an academic medical center that carries out research also strives to provide care to its immediate community. Yet, over time, the goal of serving the community may become secondary to (or be subjugated by) the research. Aligning one's own goals with one's action and having a shared purpose with other stakeholders are two separate processes, and they are not as easily achieved as one may imagine. Often, a question that is not asked in any given collaboration is, why are we all here and what do we want to accomplish?

I want to share one exercise that I use while teaching, which is a good icebreaker yet, admittedly, a bit of a setup. I ask my graduate and executive education students to divide themselves into groups and come up with a response to this question: "If we're so good, why aren't we better?" The participants endeavor to answer the question by going into details about what improvements have been missed, why there might be a certain amount of inertia in bringing about health care reform, and who might be to blame for the inertia. They really jump into this exercise and have animated conversations. Some make lists to be read out loud. When the time is up, I tell them that this twenty-minute exercise was largely futile. I get puzzled looks, but then I ask them, "Has anyone in the room defined and agreed upon what is meant by 'better'?" They all shake their heads, indicating that they have not discussed the meaning of "better." Then I go on to explain that one person's version of "better" is not my version, or necessarily that of others in that person's group.

If better for one person is higher market share, and better for me means less turnover of staff, and better for someone else is lowering costs or, in the patient's case, a higher quality of care, then we have differing views, goals, and starting points. I ask the students how we can find the shared consensus on what better means; and so the conversation on stakeholder alignment begins. The goal of stakeholder alignment is to first find common ground, before the discussions or negotiations begin; it is to make sure that we all start on the same page.

I often pull from an example of an organization I worked with to illustrate how aligned entities can both cooperate and compete with other entities while providing excellent services and quality care. The Kendal System offers a very successful set of services for aging people. Their affiliates provide continuing care, retirement communities, long-term care facilities, and nursing homes. There is also a fundraising and grant-making organization that works to support the many Kendal entities. I like to use the Kendal System as an example because it has its origins in the Quaker movement, and its affiliates are also united by a culture that asks, "How can we do this better?" They also acknowledge and foster a strong interdependence between the System's diverse entities. Within this model there is also a great amount of autonomy. The entities themselves have to balance their autonomy with a sense of shared purpose (The Kendal Corporation, 2010).

There are two reasons I like to talk about Kendal's federal-type structure. First: just like the Kendal Corporation, the health care industry is made up of entities that are both independent and interdependent. Acknowledging that health care has many independent operations with some shared goals helps one appreciate the diversity that exists within the U.S. health care industry. Second: proposing that the various stakeholders work with a federal-style model helps everyone understand that no single stakeholder unilaterally takes precedence over another. Naturally, the affiliates within the Kendal Corporation have a great advantage because they have a shared cultural sense of enhancing quality within their facilities. But even with this advantage, the idea of "better" always needs to be defined, updated, and agreed upon. An important part of the detailed ethical code that Kendal Corporation puts forward is the inherent need to place value on "participation, transparency and consensus building" (The Kendal Corporation, 2010). Consensus building is the holy grail of stakeholder alignment in the Federalist model, specifically, reaching a consensus of how "better" is defined. The steps it takes to identify "better" should never be skipped, and no constituency group should ever be left out of defining and deciding what "better" is, or what it can be.

So here we have three concepts that we will build on throughout this book. First, we have the concept of identifying stakeholders; second, we have the concept of a federal-style business approach with a shared purpose; and finally there is the concept of reaching stakeholder alignment. These are our themes, but to these we will add more ideas. We want to emphasize that stakeholder alignment only takes place when the entire group of stakeholding parties stands to benefit from the solution—a win–win, if you will. In other words, all stakeholders must see value in any given solution before they reach the ideal state of alignment. It is around these themes and ideas that we will begin to build our arguments and make our recommendations. We are not advocating for one policy change over another, and those looking for a book on health care policy will not find it here. Instead we are advocating for a way of thinking, a way of working through inevitable problems, and a way of finding middle ground or room for cooperation. And if cooperation seems impossible, we can find ways and places where co-opetition will work.

We are asking you to reflect on our examples, our stories from the trenches and the library, the realities of discord and strife in everyday stakeholder meetings in the health care setting. To some of our readers these situations may be all too familiar. Certainly, we hope the way we describe them from different stakeholders' perspectives will be refreshing and, if perhaps a little disorienting, ultimately thought provoking and useful.

1.2 THE BICKERING FAMILY

Discussions of policy reform and its implementation in health care echo throughout the halls of government these days. As these talks are ongoing, we pause to ask ourselves, what does the health care community look like to an outsider, or even to an insider? Mary Grayson, the editor of *Hospital and Health Network*, hit it on the nose: the health care world is like one huge family, whose members both love and hate one another. The family members are independent and self-righteous, yet undeniably codependant. As Grayson put it:

Being on the inside of health care is like belonging to a huge, contentious extended family where everyone is dependent on each other but at any given time someone is mad at somebody about something or other. What fun. It reminds me of my father's side of the family. They gave up the annual family reunion because in any given year so many people weren't on speaking terms with other folks that if one tried to remain neutral, it felt more like a land-mine discovery operation than a festive family event. (Grayson, 2002 p. 8)

To embrace and extend Grayson's words about the health care family and its bickering individuals, we ask you to imagine one of these annual family gatherings. Imagine that this particular family is the subject of a reality TV show, and you are the viewer. In one episode the family plans a get-together for a spring picnic where they hope to eat, soak up the sunshine, and get some exercise by playing a sport on a sprawling, grassy field. There is just one problem: no single individual can convince the others as to which sport is most enjoyable. So in the spirit of having fun, everyone brings their own sports equipment. After eating (an activity that everyone enjoys), the grandfather picks up his bat, a catcher's mitt, and a baseball. But the eldest son, an Ultimate Frisbee enthusiast, does not want to pitch baseballs to his old man. The son instead begins flinging his yellow Frisbee at his sisters, who have shown up with an assortment of lacrosse and field hockey sticks. While the sisters warm up (they actually manage to hurl balls back and forth), the spouses begin to join in. One wife has brought a rugby ball, which the grandmother, a former college cheerleader, mistakes for an American football. The grandmother looks it over and says to the young women, "I didn't know girls play football." The woman who brought the rugby ball rolls her eyes, not bothering to explain the origins of the sport and how it has caught on among college co-eds. Another spouse, a sister's husband, has brought cricket equipment; this confuses the grandfather, who has never seen such a flat-looking bat and strange-shaped catcher's mitt. Instead of asking about the bat and its purpose, the grandfather raises his own baseball bat as if challenging the young man to a duel. Occasionally, the grandfather also takes a swing at the straying Frisbee. No one is willing to call a time-out or discuss the obvious problem. The afternoon drags on with a lot of swinging, tackling, and random cheers coming from the grandmother, who believes that her good attitude just might somehow, almost miraculously, encourage everyone to cooperate.

We have allowed Mary Grayson's metaphor of a bickering family to take a fanciful turn. But what we want to describe here is an increasingly uncomfortable situation in which the stakes are very high. In our imaginary family gathering, the goal of relaxing and having fun has been replaced with the simple goal of not getting injured. Certainly, having fun seemed like a good idea at the start of the day, but with the various family members swinging bats, hurling balls and Frisbees, and tackling one another at random, the name of the game has changed. It has now become a game of survival. This is exactly what has happened in our health care world. Hospitals and physicians are just looking for ways in which to survive, while pharmaceutical companies, device manufacturers, and insurers are also expected to thrive financially. Add to this mix a not-so-well-informed patient, and we have a somewhat innocent bystander who is likely to get hurt. In other words, health outcomes have become secondary to the survival of the stakeholding entity.

> **Box 1.1** Hardin's Herdsmen
>
> A herdsman sharing a common grazing field with other herdsmen adds a single cow to his herd. He is rewarded when he sells the extra cow at the end of the season. He gains the proceeds from his original herd of cattle plus the sale of one extra cow (a +1 unit gain). However, the common grazing land is degraded by the extra grazing (a −1 unit loss). Yet the herdsman does not feel the immediate effects of the land's degradation, as it is distributed equally among him and his peers. Therefore the loss to him is a fraction of the −1 unit loss. Because of this phenomenon, all herdsmen think it a good idea to add at least one extra cow. Soon the grass does not replenish properly due to severe overgrazing, and the cattle begin to starve. With no alternative pastures, all the herdsmen are forced to abandon their dying cattle and also their livelihoods.
>
> *Source*: Hardin, G. (1968). The tragedy of the commons. *Science, 162*(5364), 1243–1248.

We want to also highlight how stakeholders have taken steps toward self-preservation, perhaps at the expense of one another and ultimately at the expense of the patient. They are often in competition with one another, but this is just the type of competing that has resulted in scenarios in which no one wins and everyone loses. This situation has often been described as the "Tragedy of the Commons," a paradox (and article title) described by Garrett Hardin (1968), a professor of human ecology. Although Professor Hardin had an almost draconian population control in mind, he was the first among his peers to explain how precious resources, if not managed correctly, would be used up. This depletion would ultimately lead to the extinction of all those depending on them (Deese, 2008). By the same token, Professor Hardin demonstrated mathematically why the stakeholders sharing in a common resource would typically be seduced by short-term gain over the long-term sustainable practices (Hardin, 1968). In Box 1.1, we explain Professor Hardin's reasoning.

While Hardin's analysis was based upon the English livestock practices of an earlier century, our examples and arguments will show that present health care is subject to the same tragedy, or possibly many tragedies.

1.3 OUR PERSPECTIVE ON STAKEHOLDER THEORY

In the health care world, the phrase *zero-sum competition* has been described by my colleagues Michael Porter and Elisabeth Olmsted Teisberg as being behind the high-cost–low-quality paradigm that has plagued health care delivery in the United States (Porter & Teisberg, 2006). Because each health care stakeholder is straining under rising costs, we often see expenses shifted from one stakeholder group to another (Dobson & Clarke, 1992; Dobson, Davanzo, & Sen, 2006). Very often stakeholders in health care may feel that a dollar lost from their pocket is a dollar gained in another entity's pocket. It is a "zero-sum competition." But what does the phrase *zero-sum* or *zero-sum competition* actually mean? Perhaps a number of our readers may have heard of game theory before. Game theory may be used to illustrate a particular situation where behavioral outcomes are measurable and easily described. Here we must be careful to make the distinction between zero-sum games and non-zero-sum games. Poker and chess are typical zero-sum games because what is lost by one player is the exact gain for the other player. Therefore the aggregate winnings taken with the aggregate loss will equal out to zero; in other words, the losses and the wins taken together sum up to zero, hence the saying zero-sum competition.

However, not all games are the same. Here we think it may be helpful to (re)visit basic game theory by extending what we have already learned from Professor Hardin's "Tragedy of the Commons," which is an example of a *non-zero-sum* game, or a competition where the outcomes do not always equal out to zero. To simplify Professor Hardin's example, let's say there are only two herders. Assume that they have come to the realization that there is merit in cooperating in order to spare the pasture land. They might then both agree not to add cattle to their herds to sustain the common resource. But as time wears on, one herder might be tempted to add one extra cow to his herd, especially if the other herder does not notice. The herders can either cooperate (we can think of them as co-competitors), or they can decide not to cooperate (noncooperators). Unlike the poker and chess players, the herdsmen play a nonzero sum game. The results of a nonzero sum game do not require one player to win and the other to lose. Both herders may win or both may lose, so the final score does not always equal zero.

Distinguishing between zero-sum competition and non-zero-sum competition is far more than a matter of semantics. It becomes important to our analysis when comparing two stakeholders vying for the same dollar to the kinds of relationships where many parties deplete common resources to everyone's detriment. For this first chapter, we need only note that the two forms of competition require different kinds of cooperation, collaborations, and alignments. Moreover, because we are dealing with several zero-sum and non-zero-sum scenarios, one solution does not fit all. In fact, the complex and fluid nature of the dysfunctional health care system requires ongoing and fluid engagement, which in turn requires that different stakeholder groups trust that other groups can think and act beyond their own narrow self-interests.

In their book *Redefining Health Care: Creating Value-Based Competition on Results*, Professors Porter and Teisberg use a delightfully illustrative metaphor of passing a "hot potato" around as costs are shifted from one stakeholder group to the next (Porter & Teisberg, 2006). To continue with that metaphor, all the stakeholders in the health care world basically end up with scorched hands. In other words, the increasing health care costs might be shifting from the employer to the provider to the insurer, and eventually back to the patient, but all the stakeholders suffer from the sting of higher costs. Yet not all the stakeholders will suffer in exactly the same way, and some might suffer more than others. Because of this asymmetry, reaching alignment can be extremely challenging. We supply you with a number of examples throughout this book, and through these examples we hope to illustrate just how complex stakeholder alignment can be. Importantly, we hope to highlight the different perspectives with which the stakeholders come to the table. You may ask whether gaining perspective will really help solve everyday challenges in health care; the answer to that question is, yes, most certainly!

We are not calling on our readers just to gain insight into the functioning of one or two different stakeholder groups; we are asking them to adopt an attitude that will allow them to envision the challenges that every stakeholder faces. We are also asking the reader to adopt an approach that facilitates cooperation, if not co-opetition with a shared goal in mind. This is a book built on pragmatism, with workable examples, case studies of stakeholder stand-offs, and tools for anticipating places where alignment might occur. Finally, we ask our readers to read through these examples, think of their own experiences, and reach their own conclusions.

1.4 THE BIRTH AND EVOLUTION OF STAKEHOLDER THEORY

How did stakeholder theory emerge, and why is it well suited to analyze the misgivings in the health care industry in the United States? Let us briefly discuss the origins of stakeholder theory and what its implications are for the U.S. health care system.

Stakeholder theory is a synthesis of thought that was first drawn together in a landmark book, *Strategic Management: A Stakeholder Approach*, by Edward R. Freeman (1984). A second book, cowritten by Freeman with two other colleagues, fleshed out the mindset and principles of ethical leadership and described how such leadership can demonstrate and explain the ways in which every key stakeholder is "better off" when a stakeholder approach is used to create value (Freeman, Harrison, & Wicks, 2007). Freeman, a professor of business administration and religious studies at the University of Virginia, drew his inspiration from his own studies in ethics as well as disparate areas of research such as psychology, operations management, and systems engineering.

Freeman's books are important because they were among the first works to adopt a systems approach to encouraging better business through improvements for all the stakeholders in any given institution or corporate enterprise. Traditional business models focused on the financiers and how to improve the return on investment for share- and stock-holding parties. Freeman found fault with this model and suggested everyone in the company's immediate ecology—the suppliers, the customers, the employees, the distributors, and all the communities that support these entities—needs to benefit in order for the company to achieve long-term sustainability. He felt that talking about increasing stockholder profit was only part of the equation (albeit critical), and that most businesses did not realize that great possibility lay in creating value for each and every stakeholding party. Freeman et al. (2007) wrote: "The beauty of capitalism is that there are multiple ways to create value for stakeholders." With that clear view of capitalism as the main elixir for cooperation between stakeholders, we will go back briefly through history, starting with how we have evolved this more robust idea of cooperation, co-opetition and sustainability through stakeholder theory. Later, we will further discuss how this all relates to health care in the United States.

We start with an essay about a pencil. In his oft-quoted essay *I Pencil: My Family Tree as Told to Leonard E. Read* (Read, 1958, 2008), the author, Leonard Read, presents the notion that no single person knows exactly how to manufacture a pencil; instead many thousands of people rely on one another in order to produce an end product that many more millions of people will use. The essay is an elegant reminder of how so many parts of such a simple item are sourced, modified, and unified into a single product, which is then shipped and delivered to the end user. Mr. Read wrote his essay to highlight the power of free-market economics. He was arguing that if a single entity, such as a government, were to orchestrate the production of a pencil, it would take such a long time and result in such a costly pencil that customers would never buy it (Read, 1958, 2008).

Milton Friedman, the late Nobel Prize–winning economist, used Mr. Read's example in a popular TV miniseries *Free to Choose*, made for PBS in the 1980s (Friedman, 1980). For many years now I have utilized a video clip from the PBS series of Professor Friedman telling the pencil story. My executive participants and graduate students typically watch with great interest and enthusiasm. Professor Friedman admires the story because it captures the notion of the invisible hand of capitalism proposed by the philosopher Adam Smith (Professor Friedman states this in an afterword added to a reprint of Mr. Read's essay) (Read, 1958, 2008). But Professor Freidman hits on one point that resonated with Mr. Read and advocates of free trade—that there is great possibility in cooperation without coercion, especially when financial incentive presents itself. Indeed, Mr. Read's essay highlights the bringing together of items produced by a diversity of countries, people, and suppliers. The production of such items can only eventuate from cooperation (Read, 1958, 2008).

In discussions following viewing of the video clip, I point out that today we are not only amazed by how cooperation works across borders when major barriers to trade and free enterprise are removed; we are also concerned, if not manically driven, by a fear that the pencil's wood is not, for example, logged from the earth's irreplaceable old-growth forests. We demand that the compounds in the graphite and the paint on the pencil's surface do not harm our children. We also hope that we can use the pencil knowing that the people assembling its pieces are treated with dignity, and that labor laws protect their basic human rights. We hope that the pencil will not leach noxious chemicals into our environment when discarded.

In summary, we want a stakeholder approach to building our pencil. We want it to meet certain standards, and we do not want to squander our precious resources on making pencils if the end result is disastrous depletion, human abuse, environmental pollution, and the poisoning of the pencil's users. In other words, we do not want a tragedy of the commons—the paradigm of short-term gain and long-term pain proposed by Hardin (1968). Paradoxically, we, the consumers, have also become pickier. We want our pencils to come in a variety of shapes, colors, and sizes. We want them to be affordable, if not half-price, because we all love a good bargain when we go shopping.

1.5 HOW HAVE WE EVOLVED SYSTEMS FOR COOPERATION AMONG STAKEHOLDERS?

Meeting all the demands of contemporary consumers takes great effort, and perhaps a bit more coordination than Read suggests in his classic essay. Manufacturers have developed methods to accommodate the needs of fastidious consumers, fast-changing trends, demanding retailers, competitors undercutting them on price, and lobby groups calling for "fair trade." Some very successful early manufacturers adopted practices that created efficiencies and eliminated waste through better coordination. Joseph Juran, William Edward Deming, and Henry Ford pioneered many of our current ideas regarding increased efficiency in the early part of the twentieth century in the United States. These ideas later spread to the rest of the world, most notably to Japan, where they were adopted and integrated into a manufacturing system by Taiichi Ohno of the Toyota Motor Corporation (Cusumano, 1988; Krafcik, 1988; Murman et al., 2002; Ohno, 1988).

In the aftermath of World War II, Mr. Ohno, a chief engineer at Toyota, was told to help his company "catch up" with U.S. car manufacturers and surpass them in as little as three years. Through careful observation, and while logging thousands of hours in practical application, Mr. Ohno achieved one of the highest productivity rates known to car manufacturers at the time. He established what became known as the "Toyota Production System," or TPS. This approach to manufacturing has since became known simply as "Lean" (Krafcik, 1988), and today it is arguably the most influential philosophy not only in manufacturing but also in a great number of process-oriented service-sector companies, and even in hospitals (Murman et al., 2002; Ohno, 1988; Womack, 1996; Womack & Jones Roos, 1990;).

One major teaching of Lean manufacturing is the philosophy that suppliers should be treated as stakeholders in the end product. Ohno believed that the suppliers of car parts had to feel that they had a stake in the final product (a finished car). Where other car manufactures haggled over price and quality issues with their suppliers, Toyota entered into long-term strategic partnerships to create quality parts that fit perfectly in their products (Murman et al., 2002). As later writers on Lean thinking observed, "value delivery is possible only when there is mutual agreement (tacit or explicit) among key stakeholders" (Murman et al., 2002, p. 9). Toyota's suppliers became guardians of the Toyota quality promise to the end users. In a case study of a new Toyota factory in Kentucky, a supplier of car seats devised production and quality-control systems to meet the criteria and high standards of its new client (Mishina, 1992). As Toyota became more successful at selling more cars to an ever-increasing market share, Toyota's stakeholders also shared in the manufacturer's success (Krafcik, 1988).

The above example of stakeholder co-opetition in manufacturing is a simple one. In that scenario there are three basic stakeholder groups: the manufacturers; the suppliers; and the end users, also known as the consumers. When talking about the U.S. health care industry, we may at times also simplify the stakeholder groups to a few, commonly known as the "four Ps"—payers, purchasers, providers, and patients. We may talk about stakeholders such as the employers, the insurers, the providers, the drug and device companies, the government, and the patients. For the sake of simplicity we may refer sometimes to commonly used language to name four major stakeholding groups. For example, in one scenario we may talk about the payers, the different types of providers, and the patients. The term "providers" covers hospitals, physicians (both independent and those belonging to umbrella groups), and specialists, and may extend to anyone providing any type of health service. It is important to note that even though hospitals and doctors both provide health services, they are very distinct stakeholding groups and often find alignment to be a great challenge. In different situations, the "payer" may be the employers purchasing the health insurance, the insurer itself, the government, or the patient. In any case, we make the particular nomenclature clear to our readers in each and every example throughout this book.

Of course, anyone working in the health care community may know that there are dozens of stakeholders in any given situation. But this fact is not always fully realized. To make this apparent, I often give another exercise to my students and executive participants: I ask them to think of all the stakeholder groups with which they work, and to make a list of nine. Many people initially question whether they can come up with such a robust list, yet once they get started they identify more than nine; they might list twenty stakeholders or more. Perhaps that is why the metaphor of health care as a dysfunctional and bickering extended family resonates so well with those of us who have worked in the field.

1.6 THE NO-LOOK PASS

Just for a moment, let us go back to our imaginary scenario of the dysfunctional family. Let us imagine that, as the day has grown long, some of the family members have exhausted themselves. They sit on the sidelines nursing their injuries. They are dishevelled, bruised, broken, angry, and sad. Even though everyone's intention was to come to a picnic and have fun playing a sport in the bright sunshine, in the end they spent the afternoon simply trying not to get hurt or minimizing the damage of an injury. The grandmother, who is not satisfied with the day's outcome, suggests that everyone try one more time to agree on a single sport. She spots a basketball court in the adjacent playground, and since not one of her family members came intending to play basketball, she manages to convince everyone that no individual will be favored if they all play that game. Reluctantly and one by one, the wounded family members slowly get up and agree to grant the grandmother her wish. They successfully divide themselves up into two teams. A basketball is borrowed from another group who have just concluded an energetic game.

The family members, now divided into teams, make strategic plans to foil one another. On one team a sister tells her brother to drop to the right, then cut into the center for the pass; he agrees that he will be there to catch the ball and take an open shot at the basket. The sister promises she will mislead her opponents by first looking left before throwing the ball in the opposite direction—a seemingly foolproof strategy of a no-look pass. However, when the play begins the ball is bounced to the sister, and the plan fails miserably. The brother is slow to fake to the left, and he gets successfully blocked by his opponent, his wife. The sister fails to improvise and does not notice that her father-in-law is free and cutting left; instead she hurls the basketball to center court without even looking for her brother. The ball bounces a couple of times and then rolls out of bounds. The no-look pass might have worked had the siblings had more time to practice the offensive play, but with little coordination they had little hope for success.

This scenario brings us to a closing point about stakeholders and health care. Those of us who work in the health care world are well aware that cooperation alone is not the only component of successfully caring for patients. What we need, but are often lacking, is a continued and sustained coordination effort. At the moment, coordination between different stakeholding parties is fraught with failed (albeit well-meaning) no-look passes. Different types of providers often hand patients off to one another with little coordination; insurers often reject claims, seemingly arbitrarily, merely because some piece of information may be missing (or mistyped), costing precious time and money in reprocessing. Patients often sabotage their own health by not following or understanding appropriate health advice, or by not complying with prescriptions, diets, or suggested exercise regimens. There are an unlimited number of examples of missed no-look passes.

Here we get to the heart of why this is not a policy book. Our health care is under great scrutiny at the moment, and changes are afoot. Change comes in many forms; it comes as part of a mandate, such as The Health Care and Education Reconciliation Act of 2010, and also from enterprise-driven initiatives. Yet, whatever changes are implemented or rejected, we need a much-improved mindset in order to clearly understand and cooperate with each and every stakeholding party. When we talk about better coordination in health care, we are not referring only to better and more descriptive medical electronic records for tracking patients (although that may well be one part of gaining value); we are talking about a universal coordination of ethical values, of qualities that will guarantee better value for all stakeholding parties and, most importantly, better health outcomes for the population as a whole. Creating real value for all stakeholders is central to stakeholder theory, and using Lean principles can offer one tried and true structure for achieving these goals. We close this chapter with one last quote from a book important for its writing on the creation of value through Lean teachings. We have split the quote into two parts to allow you, the reader, a moment to think about the first statement before moving on to the second part of the quote.

Academia often concentrates on data collection and analysis; industry members are more interested in "how to" guides; and government members, with their contractual mindsets, are most concerned with program deliverables, schedules and cost reduction.... (Murman et al., 2002, p. 9)

While the authors of this quote are referring to the aeronautics industry, quite surprisingly, it may also resonate with our health care world. How would you characterize the stakeholders you interact with everyday? Where do they place the most emphasis in their day-to-day dealings with you and others? Importantly, do you look to match expectations before attempting to find a solution to a problem? Here is the second half of the quote:

Forging a structure and a method of operation that engage each member group is essential to delivering value to all. The matching of expectations to capabilities among all stakeholders is a lesson that applies at any level of the enterprise. (Murman et al., 2002, p. 9)

Because of some seemingly contradictory goals and cultures, it would appear that the stakeholders in the health care world are bound to clash repeatedly and calamitously. I spoke to Thomas Jones, a chief negotiator for a large health system on the East Coast. He described his negotiations with payers as nothing less than contentious. He put it this way: "We have fundamental conflicts in our goals." Jones was speaking about one particular medium-sized employer that wanted better rates for its employees to control rising health care costs. Yet this corporation was not willing to align expectations with what the provider was able to offer; as Mr. Jones put it, "they want everything and promise nothing in exchange."

What we are suggesting for a negotiation—be it over cost or performance, or both—is to actually invite all the players to have a seat at the table very early on in the process. When a high-performing manufacturer designs a product under Lean principles, all the stakeholders are present. This would include, for example, the materials and part suppliers, the workers that build and assemble the product, the end users, and, of course, the designers. This process is sometimes called *onboarding*, a step that is baked into my model for project management in health care. These groups are not just niche players—they are responsible for the end product. They are holding a stake in the end product. We have found that stakeholder onboarding and engaging all the parties early and often, rather than later and infrequently, add up to a very effective strategy for the value-creation process. This first step helps in identifying all the stakeholders from the starting point to the ending point, not just the ones relevant to one particular stage of the game. It is only after establishing who all the stakeholders are that we may move on to bringing greater value to health care, and to delivering better health outcomes.

REFERENCES

Boudreau, K.J., & Lakhani, K.R. (2009). How to manage outside innovation: should external innovators be organized in collaborative communities or competative markets? The answer depends on three crucial issues. *Sloan Management Review*, 50(4), 69–76.

Cusumano, M. A. (1988). Manufacturing innovation: Lessons from the Japanese auto industry. *Sloan Management Review* 30(1), 29–39.

Deese, R. S. (2008). A metaphor at midlife: "The tragedy of the commons" turns 40. *Endeavour*, 32(4), 152–155.

Dobson, A, & Clarke, R.L. (1992). Shifting no solution to problem of increasing costs. *Healthcare Financial Management*, 46(7), 24–28, 22–33.

Dobson, A., J. Davanzo, et al. (2006). The cost-shift payment 'hydraulic': foundation, history, and implications. *Health Affairs* 25(1), 22–33.

Freeman, E. R. (1984). *Strategic management: A stakeholder approach*. Boston, MA: Pitman.

Freeman, E. R., Harrison, J. S., & Wicks, A. C. (2007). *Managing for stakeholders: survival, reputation and success*. New Haven, CT: Yale University Press.

Fisher, L.M. (1992, March 29). Preaching love thy competitor. *New York Times*, p. 1–6.

Friedman, M. (Writer) (1980). Power of the market [Television series episode]. In M. Latham, R. Chitester, & M. Peacock (Producers), *Free to choose*. USA: PBS.

Grayson, M. (2002). Three legs. *Hospitals & Health Networks, 76*, 8.

Hardin, G. (1968). The tragedy of the commons. *Science, 162*(5364), 1243–1248.

Keller, K. L. (2008). *Best practice cases in branding*, 3rd ed. Upper Saddle River, NJ: Pearson Prentice-Hall.

The Kendal Corporation. (2010). *Questions and answers about the Kendal System*. Retrieved from http://www.kendal.org/about/QADocuments.aspx

Krafcik, J. F. (1988). Triumph of the lean production system. *Sloan Management Review, 30*(1), 41–52.

Mishina, K. (1992). Toyota Motor Manufacturing, USA Inc. HBS No. 0-693-019. Boston, MA: Harvard Business School Publishing.

Murman, E., Allen, T., Bozdogan, K., Cutcher-Gershenfeld, J., McManus, H., Nightingale, D., et al. (2002). *Lean enterprise value: Insights from MIT's lean aerospace initiative*. New York, NY: Palgrave.

Ohno, T. (1988). Toyota production system: Beyond large-scale production. *New York, Productivity Press*.

Porter, M. E., & Teisberg, E. O. (2006). *Redefining health care: Creating value-based competition on results*. Boston, MA: Harvard Business School Press.

Read, L. E. (1958, 2008). *I, Pencil. My family tree as told to Leonard E. Read* (50th Anniversary ed.). Irvington-on-Hudson, NY: The Foundation for Economic Education, Inc.

Womack, J. P. and D. T. Jones (1996). Lean thinking: Banish waste and create wealth in your corporation. *New York, Free Press*.

Womack, J.P., Jones, D.T., & Roos, D. (1990). The machine that changed the world: the story of lean production. New York: Rawson Associates.

2 The Gordian Knot

2.1 WHAT WE GET FOR THE DOLLARS WE SPEND HERE IN THE UNITED STATES

In this chapter we want to look at the value in health care here in the United States: "If we're so good, why aren't we better?" In Chapter 1 I explained how we use this question as a set-up for emerging and existing health care leaders to help them see, firsthand, how defining "better" brings many different answers from a diversity of stakeholders working in the health care arena. However, if we want to get an idea about the overall performance of the United States as far as health care is concerned, what question or questions do we ask? A good place to start is to ask how we evaluate the value delivered to patients in the United States.

"Value" is a concept that is often bandied around without much description as to what is meant by the word. Specifically, health care analysts use the word "value" to connote a push–pull dynamic between three major challenges. We use the analogy of the Iron Triangle to highlight these challenges as cost, quality, and access; these are placed at the points on the Iron Triangle depicted in Figure 2.1. The triangle is a good pictorial tool because it also depicts the trade-offs between cost, quality, and access. This may sound familiar, as many companies and organizations have adopted similar Iron Triangles to describe the trade-offs they face in delivering a product or service to their customers. A variation on this and other Iron Triangles was used by my colleague Regina Hertzlinger to connote how Congress, insurers, and hospitals interact in the delivery of health care (Manhattan Institute for Policy Research, 2007).

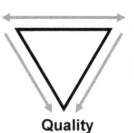

Cost

Rising costs
Increasing numbers of users are priced out of health care. Those who can afford health care must pay more to subsidize the nonpayers.

Access

Decreasing access
As access decreases, providing consistency in care becomes impossible.

Quality

Falling quality
As costs rise, insurers and providers are further challenged in providing quality care.

FIGURE 2.1 The Iron Triangle.

The Iron Triangle tool is useful, but I always fear we are oversimplifying. It describes these trade-offs, but alone it is not really enough to make a solid argument. We must also review the literature to show where value is eroded in the U.S. health care market. Traditionally, we start by comparing our health outcomes and the cost of health care delivery with those of our peers. So, who is in our peer group? They are countries with similar levels of economic achievement and academic might. They are places that have already gone through many of the awkward growing pains that developing countries face. Typically, they are places run by a democracy, with liberalized economies free of major corruption, and possessing a free press and an uninhibited culture of research and technological development. We are usually compared to countries such as Canada, the United Kingdom, Australia, Japan, France, and Germany, to name just a few.

But when we compare ourselves to our peers, our health care does not produce the health outcomes we may expect. This trend is not new. A number of important health indicators measuring performance show we have fallen behind our peers. So what are the indicators typically used to benchmark health care? An oft-quoted World Health Organization (WHO) report published in 2000 ranked U.S. health care's performance 72nd out of 191 nations (WHO, 2000). The countries were ranked on a measure that plots health outcomes (such as access to care, equity of care, and preventative medicine) as a function of health resources (Jamison & Sandbu, 2001; WHO, 2000). Put simply, this measure takes into account our relative income levels, so the playing field is leveled and we can see what we can achieve given our resources (Jamison & Sandbu, 2001). In this WHO ranking, the United States is behind places such as Sri Lanka, China, and Mexico. And we are far from the top ten countries, which include economically advanced nations such as Spain, France, and Japan. Critics of this report say that this measure is flawed, as it does not accurately portray the achievements that are better captured by simply comparing health outcomes (Jamison & Sandbu, 2001; Organisation for Economic Co-operation and Development [OECD], 2010). After all, we do have far better health outcomes than both China and Mexico, as well as a great number of other countries that rank ahead of the United States in that 2000 WHO report.

Traditional health indicators measure outcomes such as infant mortality, life expectancy at birth, maternal mortality ratio, and deaths that could have been prevented given timely access to quality care (sometimes referred to as amenable mortality). Comparing these and other indicators across countries can tell a story about the quality of health care available. The fact that the U.S. infant mortality rate is higher than those of other developed countries year after year means that we lag behind places we would like to compare ourselves with—countries such as Canada, the United Kingdom, and Australia (OECD, 2010). Another indicator, the maternal mortality ratio, examines the maternal death rate associated with 100,000 live births and is a marker for risk of death related to pregnancy—or, as some might explain, the obstetric risk directly related to the quality of prenatal, birthing, and postnatal care. The U.S. risk level is above the high-income average. In fact, the United States is one of the worst performers among the world's wealthy nations. In this instance, we are more on par with countries such as the Republic of Moldova and Slovakia (WHO, 2008).

The Organisation for Economic Co-operation and Development (OECD) tracks a vast number of economic and health indicators across thirty developed nations. One important indicator is the overall life expectancy (LE) at birth, which has increased substantially in all wealthy nations over the past few decades. The OECD country average is approximately seventy-nine years. The United States' LE is 77.9, which is below that average (OECD, 2010). At first pass, the United States' LE may not seem too far removed from the average, but if you study the OECD chart (Figure 2.2) you can see how the United States arrives in the bottom half of the participating countries. Consider the fact that Canada's LE at birth is 80.7, France's is almost 81, and Japan's is 82 (OECD, 2010). We see that there is a wider gap between the United States and countries with particularly strong and diverse economies like our own. In 1964, Japan and the United States have an identical life expectancy at birth (70.3; OECD, 2010). The question have becomes, why in the past 30 years has the United States not made gains similar to those of other industrialized nations despite greater spending on health care?

Several other country surveys inform us that the United States is falling behind its peers. This is especially true when looking at a comparative study of preventable deaths in the populations of people age 74 and under, living in the world's top nineteen economically developed nations. These surveys show that the United States made only tiny inroads into reducing the mortality rate caused by treatable conditions such as diabetes, cardiovascular disease, and some cancers. The United States ranked last on the list, revealing a preventable death rate of about 115 per 100,000 people in the yearlong study period from 2003 to 2004. That rate is far higher than Canada's preventable death rate, which stood at 77 per 100,000 people in that same time frame. The study concluded that between 75,000 and 101,000 lives may have been saved in the twelve-month survey period had those patients had access to quality health care (Nolte & McKee, 2008).

The next question is why this might be the case. A study of chronically ill adults in eight developed nations pointed to vast discrepancies in access, safety, and efficacy of health care received by patients residing in the United States

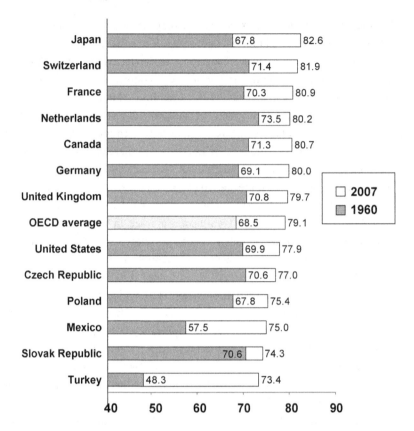

FIGURE 2.2 Life expectancy at birth in select Organisation for Economic Co-operation and Development [OECD] countries. OECD average based on all OECD country data available for that year. Canada data unavailable for 1960; 1961 data were used. Adapted from *OECD health data 2010* by the Organisation for Economic Co-operation and Development, 2010. Available at www.oecd.org/health/healthdata.

(Schoen, Osborn, How, Doty, & Peugh, 2009). In short, this survey looked at three major aspects of care: problems related to accessing care due to costs, problems in the coordination of care, and errors in care (this includes problems with retrieving lab reports or records in timely fashion). The United States consistently came last in a ranking that evaluated all three of these areas separately (Schoen et al.).

Despite these troublesome health outcomes and statistics, our health expenditure is the world's highest. On average in 2007, we spent a startling $7,290 per capita (OECD, 2010). That is not to say that each person has this much money to spend on health care; rather, it is a crude average of total spending divided by the aggregate population. The proportion of our gross domestic product (GDP) devoted to health care spending was approximately 16% by recent estimates; in Figure 2.3 we can see just how much of an outlier the United States actually is in relation to its peers (OECD, 2010). Germany, Switzerland, and France spend roughly 10% to 11% of their GDP on health care, but those countries also have better health outcomes (OECD, 2010).

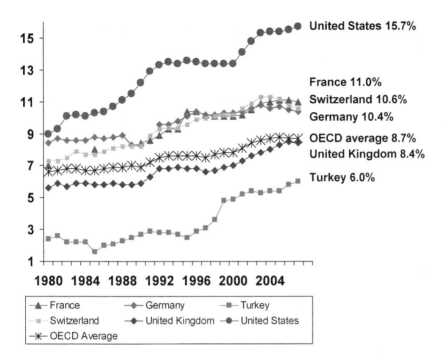

FIGURE 2.3 Total expenditures on health as a percentage of gross domestic product. The United States spends more on health—$7,290 per capita in 2007—than any other country. This is almost two and a half times greater than the OECD average of $2,984 (adjusted for purchasing-power parity). Adapted from *OECD health data 2010* by the Organisation for Economic Co-operation and Development, 2010. Available at www.oecd.org/health/healthdata.

Let us look at the number of hospital beds serving our population as another measure. In the United States there are 3.2 beds per 1,000 people. In Japan, there are about 14 beds per 1,000 people, and in France and Germany there are about 7 and 8 beds per 1,000 people, respectively (OECD, 2010). However, Japan and France report per-capita health spending more in line with the OECD average of $2,984 (OECD, 2010). Despite our lead in spending on health care, Americans get far fewer doctor consultations per annum (about four) than the number of average doctor visits in other OECD nations (OECD, 2010).

Let us compare the United States to the United Kingdom. These two nations have similar disease burdens, income gaps, and diversity in terms of ethnicity and age. Certainly we might conclude that we are roughly on par with them. But perhaps unlike the United Kingdom, we also have a capacity to spend more on each person (OECD, 2010). Indeed, this is seen as an advantage. Yet the United Kingdom spends roughly half the amount of money the United States spends on each patient in a typical year and still gets better results as far as health outcomes are concerned. It is all too easy to point the finger at one stakeholder group over another and blame one group for value erosion; but that is not what this book is about, and there is no value in assigning blame. We need to ask not only why our system has not produced the same value as other comparably rich nations, but also who the players are in our health system and how they are dealing with the erosion of value. The answer to these questions lies in the examination of the constituencies that hold the stakes in the U.S. health care environment.

The Iron Triangle presented in Figure 2.1 touches on only some of the major issues facing health care delivery in the United States; perhaps it is a good model, if only to demonstrate the simplest of dynamics between the three major issues: cost, access, and quality. Over the years I have begun to suggest a preferred model that also introduces a fourth variable—stakeholder satisfaction—and replaces "access" with "coverage." These days we suggest that the shape of health care delivery is not a triangle; instead it is more like a knotted rope. We introduce you to the Gordian knot—a knot that is so complex it seems impossible to untie. This is an analogy we will pick up later in this chapter once we have reviewed the literature.

2.2 WHAT ARE THE MAJOR COST-INFLATORS?

Some of the cost drivers for U.S. health care are pretty obvious. We have an aging population, and the older the population gets, the more costly medical attention it needs and, therefore, the higher the cost of caring for this subpopulation (Keehan et al., 2008). The second thing is that within this aging population there is a bulge of baby boomers hitting retirement now and in coming years. We expect them to live a little longer than previous generations, but they will not necessarily be healthier. A recent survey suggests that age influences how well people take care of themselves: baby boomers are 3.5 times more likely than the previous generation (the so-called silent generation) to postpone seeking medical attention because of costs (Thomson Reuters Healthcare, 2009).

Typical baby boomers under the age of 65 may worry about health costs because they are not yet eligible for Medicare. Instead, they are relying on employer-provided private health insurance, are privately self-insured, or have partial or no health insurance whatsoever. Some, of course, may rely on other government-funded programs such as Medicaid or health services provided to veterans and members of the military. However, a great number of privately insured baby boomers have seen their health insurance premiums skyrocket in the past twenty years which, for many people, led to declines in coverage. In fact, during the 1990s, about one-half of the decline in coverage rates was directly attributable to increases in private health insurance premiums (Chernew, Cutler, & Keenan, 2005). This trend may be accelerating in recent times, as the economic recession has seen the number of privately insured persons dwindle (Cohen, 2010).

In the United States, almost everyone over the age of 65 is eligible for Medicare (Colamery, 2003), so we know that spending has begun and will continue to strain Medicare (Edlund, Lufkin, & Franklin, 2003). This trend is well underway, as the bulk of baby boomers are reaching retirement age now and the young population is making up a smaller proportion of the U.S. population (Centers for Disease Control and Prevention [CDC], 2007; Edlund, Lufkin, & Franklin, 2003). Medicare is based on a traditional entitlement model (Centers for Medicare and Medicaid Services [CMS], 2005), meaning that younger, healthier people pay for the benefits of the older, sicker population through federal and state revenues that come from taxes (Colamery, 2003). If the older population is much greater in number and sicker than the younger population, or if the ratio between young and old continues to shift, the system becomes prone to financial collapse (Martin & Weaver, 2005). By 2030 the number of Americans aged 65 and older is expected to make up about 20% of the population; that is roughly 71 million people—a more than twofold jump in the number of those currently eligible for Medicare in the United States (CDC, 2007; Thomson Reuters Healthcare, 2009).

In addition to these long-term strains on government-sponsored health insurance, the economic downturn and subsequent recession has had a detrimental effect on many people's ability to afford health coverage before the retirement age. As jobs get cut, many former employees lose their private health insurance (Sack & Zezima, 2009; Thomson Reuters Healthcare, 2009). Medicaid, a program jointly funded by federal and state governments which provides medical assistance to low-income families and individuals who do not have private (employer-sponsored) health insurance (CMS, 2005), saw a surge in new enrollees in 2008. A recent survey reported enrollment spikes as high as 10% in some states by the end of 2008 (Sack & Zezima, 2009).

Importantly, these increases are often well beyond what many states expected. In the state of Florida, officials reported just over a 10% jump in the twelve-month period ending in November 2008—the highest increase seen since the program was implemented (Sack & Zezima, 2009). While the federal government picks up a little over half of the Medicaid expense (about 57%), the states have traditionally covered the rest. Paradoxically, just as many states become less able to afford the government-sponsored program due to falling tax revenues, the demand for such services increases (Sack & Zezima, 2009).

Hospitals and medical practices both large and small argue that because reimbursements made through Medicare and, particularly, Medicaid are at or below the true cost of care, the unpaid portion of those costs must be passed on to private payers (employers and consumers using private health insurance) (America's Health Insurance Plans [AHIP], 2008; Dobson, Davanzo, & Sen, 2006). This issue has also been dubbed the "cost-shift payment hydraulic," a phrase that captures the notion that hospitals use funds from private payers to cover activities that also align with specific hospitals' missions (Dobson et al., 2006). Insurers and providers have hired outside actuaries to look into this so-called cost shift. One such recent consultant's report concluded that commercial payers absorb about $88.8 billion every year in extra costs because of growing shortfalls in Medicare and Medicaid reimbursements (Fox & Pickering, 2008).

In reality, this measurement simply represents the payment-level differences between Medicare, Medicaid, and the commercial payers; it does not estimate the true cost that is shifted to the commercial payers. The actual amount may be lower or even higher, depending on a number of factors. To shift costs successfully to private payers, a provider typically has a certain amount of market power (Dobson et al., 2006). In addition, hospitals can raise funds through donations to help cover shortfalls. But providers also need to absorb the costs of uninsured patients who cannot pay at all, in addition to the shortfall in payment from Medicaid and Medicare patients (Fox & Pickering, 2008). However, "safety net" hospitals that serve a large population of uninsured or government-insured patients may be eligible for extra government funding through the disproportionate-share hospital (DSH) program. It is important to note that this government program has seen a number of reincarnations over the years and may face cuts or total elimination due to recommendations by the Congressional Budget Office or the Centers for Medicare and Medicaid Services (Spivey & Kellermann, 2009).

To summarize, the shrinking pool of private payers face ever-increasing costs because fewer can afford to absorb the shortfalls in costs from a ballooning pool of publicly funded consumers. When we put the issues of our aging population, cost shifting, and the current economic crisis aside, we must still note that other factors such as the rise in obesity and changes in lifestyle have caused a shift in the disease burden. This is a long-term trend that formed over the past 100 years, and it is also related to the fact that threats from many infectious diseases and dangerous working conditions have been abated. In the past thirty years, it has become clear that chronic diseases have replaced acute diseases as the leading cause of morbidity and death. Furthermore, the long-term care of chronically ill patients is a major healthcare cost driver (Edlund et al., 2003). Chronic illnesses in the aging population include, but are not limited to, problems such as cancer, hypertension, and skeletal problems like rheumatism (CDC, 2007). Because Medicare came to fruition when acute care was a larger cost, Medicare alone cannot absorb the costs of the long-term care and custodial services typically needed by chronically ill and aging patients (Edlund et al., 2003).

Problems like asthma and diabetes have also increased over the past few decades in the United States. These are chronic conditions that, in many instances, have little to do with aging. Obesity is another major health problem that contributes to the onset of a vast number of chronic conditions. Many obese patients often have not one but numerous, chronic comorbidities influencing their health outcomes, life expectancy, and overall quality of life (Finkelstein, Fiebelkorn, & Wang, 2003; Finkelstein, Trogdon, Cohen, & Dietz, 2009). Recent estimates indicate that annual medical spending related to obesity had hit $147 billion by 2008. The figure has increased from an annual $78.5 billion in spending by 1998 estimates (Finkelstein et al., 2003; Finkelstein et al., 2009). Figure 2.4 contains a chart reflecting the costs attributed to obesity.

As America becomes fatter—and all evidence suggests we are still getting fatter (Franco Sassi, Cecchini, & Rusticelli, 2009)—the incidence of type 2 diabetes is going to increase further, along with cardiovascular issues, gallbladder disease, and a number of cancers associated with being overweight (WHO, 2009). To complicate matters, lapses in treatment of chronic conditions like type 2 diabetes can ultimately drive health care costs higher. For example, there is strong evidence that many diabetics experiencing gaps in routine care (due to a lapse in Medicaid coverage) face higher treatment costs down the road (Hall, Harman, & Zhang, 2008). This is true, as a diabetic may be forced to visit an emergency department when a simple health problem that should have needed only minor attention goes untreated and becomes more complicated.

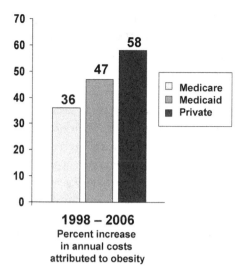

FIGURE 2.4 Health care spending attributable to obesity. Adapted from "Annual medical spending attributable to obesity: Payer-and service-specific estimates" by E. A. Finkelstein, J. G. Trogdon, J. W. Cohen, & W. Dietz, 2009, *Health Affairs, 28*(5), w822–w831. Finkelstein et al.'s calculations are based on data from the 1998 and 2006 Medical Expenditure Panel Survey.

Asthma is another strong example of a chronic condition showing a multiplier effect on the costs of treatment when not managed properly. In this case, treatment inequities have profound effect on costs and disparities of health outcomes, especially among minorities and the poor (Wright, 2006). As with many chronic diseases, the exact etiology of asthma in the United States is somewhat elusive and therefore difficult to stamp out. Rises in asthma prevalence have been ascribed to everything from Cesarean birthing to the timing of birth in the autumn months (Roduit et al., 2009; Wu et al., 2008). Developing nations of lesser economic means than the United States are also seeing large increases in asthma, perhaps related to environmental factors that trigger asthma, such as rising pollution and tobacco use (WHO, 2008). However, within the borders of the United States, we are also seeing very different treatment trajectories (Moorman et al., 2007) that result in suboptimal outcomes.

We know from national surveys that white children suffering from asthma have more visits with a physician in an office setting compared to black children with asthma, who are more likely to end up in a hospital setting like an emergency room (ER; Moorman et al., 2007). Treatment in hospitals, especially in the ER (or emergency department, sometimes abbreviated as ED), may very well be a lot more expensive for the system than regular physician visits in cases where asthma is more appropriately managed. This is because many children with asthma get less than optimal care in the ED setting (Cavazos Galvan, 2006). Proper management may include prescription and training in the use of inhalers, which can mitigate and sometimes completely prevent the onset of life-threatening asthma attacks (Peppe, Mays, Chang, Becker, & DiJulio, 2007).

Patients who return to the ED multiple times with poorly managed chronic conditions also contribute to ED crowding (Hoot & Aronsky, 2008; Pham, Patel, Millin, Kirsch, & Chanmugam, 2006), a problem that typically increases hospitals' operational costs. ED crowding, which is both a consequence of and a driver for health cost inflation, has many contributing factors (Newton, Keirns, Cunningham, Hayward, & Stanley, 2008). ED visits increased by 26% to 28% between 1992 and 2005 (Weber et al., 2008), yet the number of EDs dropped by 9% (Kellermann, 2006). While EDs serve the obvious purpose of treating trauma cases, they are also the only place where patients can seek urgent (but not necessarily emergency) after-hours care. Kellerman's 2006 article in the *New England Journal of Medicine* traces ED closures to the 1986 Emergency Medical Treatment and Labor Act, which mandated that everyone residing in the United States must have the legal right to emergency care, regardless of the ability to pay for the care provided. The closures are a consequence, according to Kellerman, of the unsustainable cost burden from providing care to nonpaying health consumers.

Perhaps it is surprising to find that the proportion of uninsured patients accepted into EDs in the United States remained relatively steady (between 16.1% and 14.5%) over the past three decades. Importantly, the demographic that started visiting EDs in greater numbers is persons with family income equivalent to or greater than 400% of the federal poverty level (Weber et al., 2008). In other words, middle-income individuals are using the ED in increasing numbers. So what is happening? Part of this trend may be related to decreasing access, which in many cases is related to higher deductibles. We know that since the 1990s employers have been shifting costs to employees by sponsoring less health coverage (Chernew et al., 2005). No doubt for many working professionals with little coverage or no benefits whatsoever, small health problems go unchecked until they require urgent attention in an ED.

For many patients, it may be easier to go to an ED that must treat them than to find a primary care physician who is convenient and willing to take Medicaid. Indeed, being uninsured and/or poor is strongly correlated to ED visits for health problems better suited to primary care (Begley, Vojvodic, Seo, & Burau, 2006). Access, however, is not related only to lack of health insurance coverage. Another aspect of access has more to do with finding physicians willing to take any new patients at all (Hall, Lemak, Steingraber, & Schaffer, 2008).

Much has been written about the severe shortage of primary care specialists in the United States. Simply finding a primary care specialist who accepts Medicaid, offers accessible office hours and a short waiting time to get an appointment, and is accessible by public transportation may be increasingly difficult (Hall, Lemak et al., 2008). Some suggest that fewer medical students can afford to go into primary care because they will struggle to meet the financial obligations of student loans when they start practicing (Spellman, 2008). One possible explanation is that many medical students choose instead to specialize in an area that is more lucrative, thus securing a promise of financial stability after accumulating years' worth of debt in medical school (Spellman).

Unfortunately, one very dangerous outcome of ED crowding includes hospitals' having to divert ambulances to other providers that may be further away. Figures from a survey showed that diversions occurred about half a million times over the course of a single year (Kellermann, 2006). Another aspect of ED crowding relates to poorer expectations of care and satisfaction—concepts that we will tackle specifically in the next chapter.

One area that we have not touched on yet is the administrative costs that different types of providers face in doing business with insurers. A paper published in mid-2009 attempted to tease apart the administrative costs for physicians. On aggregate, the study estimated that the work hours used by physicians and their staff to do administrative tasks added up to between $23 billion and $31 billion dollars annually (Casalino et al., 2009). The authors also noted that interactions with insurers could also benefit the delivery of medicine in terms of cost-reductions, and adherence to quality of care guidelines (Casalino et al.). Papers published by two health rights advocates and academics, Steffie Woolhandler and David Himmelstein, evaluated hospitals' administrative costs in the early 1990s and estimated that they often accounted for more than a quarter of their total costs (Woolhandler & Himmelstein, 1997; Woolhandler, Himmelstein, & Lewontin, 1993). They also noted that for-profit hospitals had particularly high administrative costs, approaching 35% of their total costs (Woolhandler & Himmelstein, 1997). The authors compared U.S. health care administrative costs to those in Canada (Woolhandler, Campbell, & Himmelstein, 2004) and concluded that a lot of value is eroded when U.S. providers interact with multiple payers, because the administrative costs consume so much capital (Himmelstein & Woolhandler, 1986, 1989, 1993; Woolhandler, Campbell, & Himmelstein, 2003; Woolhandler et al., 2004; Woolhandler & Himmelstein, 1991, 1994, 1995, 1997, 1999; Woolhandler et al., 1993).

A response to these works in the *New England Journal of Medicine* questions the appropriateness of comparing administrative costs in the United States with such costs in Canada. The article raises many valid points, including that it is technically difficult to correctly assess the true costs of administration in two countries in an isolated moment in time (Aaron, 2003). It is an understatement to write that there is a lot of disagreement as to how the administrative costs of doing business with multiple payers influence cost, quality, and access to health care delivery. We can say only that each stakeholder comes to the table with his or her own perspective on having multiple payers sponsor health care. As anyone who has taken my classes or participated in my workshops knows, I am fond of pointing out that where you stand on any given issue depends on where you sit. I insist that each participant preface all remarks by sharing his or her name, title, and organization every time he or she makes a comment. This is because I often find that the comments from an individual are a reflection of the stakeholder he or she represents or is working for.

We have talked about some of the obvious price inflators in health-related costs, many of which are not entirely unique to the United States. Specifically, the increases in chronic disease and the rising numbers in the aging population are trends that started over sixty years ago, and which bring problems that also plague other wealthy countries. Cost-shifting and the subsequent squeeze on physicians, hospitals, medical practices, and payers both public and private may be problems that are further aggravated by the economic downturn and budgetary constraints. As a consequence, hospitals in the United States may face additional operating costs generated from increasingly crowded EDs. These are just a few compelling examples of newer, more volatile homegrown cost trends that are worth following with close attention in coming years.

2.3 BETTER, NEWER, AND MORE PROMISING TECHNOLOGY: ARE ALL THE ADVANCES ADVANTAGES?

In Section 2.2 we wrote about some price inflators that are difficult to control but easy to measure in terms of growing morbidity and incidence rates. In this section we talk about costs that are easier to control but harder to measure precisely. Many care providers are not only providing treatment to patients but also competing for health consumers who are both discerning and impressionable. So how can the many types of hospitals, physicians, and medical practices promise to offer the best care and attract patients, preferably ones that come with largely funded health benefits and/or personal funds to pay in full? The variety of providers, provider organizations, pharmaceutical companies, and medical-device companies invest heavily in marketing and what is often euphemistically called "patient education." In contrast to many other countries, in the United States, direct-to-consumer marketing is legal. Marketing is not limited to advertorials and commercials—it may also include purchasing and using the latest technology to instill a sense of confidence and, ultimately, to attract more patients.

For example, to compete with other care facilities, a hospital might purchase a new type of "open" magnetic resonance imaging (MRI) machine. The traditional MRI is generally a tube that often gives patients a great sense of claustrophobia as they lie almost entirely enclosed in the unit. But an open machine looks wider and less coffin-like, and is positioned mainly over the portion of the body that needs to be imaged. However, the cost of an open MRI machine is greater than the traditional variety. The unit may be ideal for obese patients, young children (who can undergo the scan with their parents standing right next to them), and patients with anxiety about being in a mostly enclosed space (Janney, 2007). The drawback is that the new technology may not always be used in situations where it is absolutely necessary, such as on patients who do not have special needs. Not surprisingly, product information on the open MRI focuses on the more positive patient experience, such as one write-up that offered purchasers of the new machine a "comprehensive marketing approach . . . to help consumers identify InSight affiliated sites" (InSight Health Corp., 2009).

The above is a classic example of what has been dubbed the "med-tech arms race" or "medical arms race" (Luft et al., 1988). It is a race to attract more potential paying customers by offering a more comfortable patient experience, or at least the perception of an easier visit through cutting-edge technology, which may or may not be absolutely necessary. It can also be considered an example of direct marketing to a patient's sense of vulnerability. With that said, it is easy to see why the cost of care is increasing for everyone because the cost of individual patient treatment (and patient comfort) is increasing. Some might argue that a number of hospitals have gambled on the old notion, "If you build it, they will come."

But this does not happen only with new technology; existing technology can also drive up costs and be used inappropriately. The increase in the use of traditional MRI, ultrasound, nuclear medicine, computed tomography, and, in far fewer cases, radiography (X-ray) has been well documented in recent years (Smith-Bindman, Miglioretti, & Larson, 2008). Critics say the trend is due in part to a trend of overuse that does not necessarily enhance patient diagnosis, and which could also be potentially dangerous, particularly for tests that expose patients to radiation (Brenner & Hall, 2007). Others hotly contest these assertions. Several years ago Congress asked the Government Accountability Office (GAO) to evaluate the rise in imaging use and costs to Medicare (GAO, 2008). The GAO reported that spending on imaging more than doubled between 2000 and 2006, but also that private payers had already noted this and sought to curb imaging overuse.

Furthermore, the increases were specifically linked to imaging conducted in physicians' offices, yet the amount of imaging varied by region, suggesting that a portion of the imaging was inappropriate (GAO, 2008). Other academic studies pointed to similar findings, with one study showing clearly that physician self-referral and the prevalence of independent diagnostic facilities (centers outside of hospitals) were contributing to the increased imaging utilization. In other words, some physicians in the study had financial incentives to prescribe imaging, as they also held a stake in the machine or facility providing the imaging (Mitchell, 2008). Health analysts have long argued that the overuse of imaging is an example of how many doctors are prompted to practice "defensive" medicine rather than evidence-based medicine. The argument is that doctors fear losing time and money with litigious patients, so they may order more tests than necessary (Studdert et al., 2005). Yet doctors may also order redundant or unnecessary tests because patients specifically ask for a test, or because their patients may gain peace of mind from receiving negative test results (Mendelson & Carino, 2005). The notion of the doctor wanting to provide tailored care has also been cited as a reason some physicians do not adhere strictly to clinical guidelines when administering diagnostic tests and treatments (Mendelson & Carino).

Tailoring care cannot be evaluated purely in the negative light of adding costs to care. Tailored care is a complex issue when it comes to many areas of medicine—especially, for example, cancer care. Adopting newer drugs and devices when less is known about them may increase cost, but it might also decrease disease burden, suffering, or both. It may seem fair to conclude, with good evidence from clinical trials, that the newer drugs should supplant older drugs when possible, despite cost. Making the case for adopting newer technology or for sticking with older, generic drugs because of price and/or known efficacy/side effects is not always so simple.

For example, the 25-year-old generic drug tamoxifen treats women with hormone-receptor-positive breast cancer for a five-year period at a price of about $500 (Pollack, 2008). However, sometimes a woman on tamoxifen may develop resistance to the drug, a problem that can open the door to a return of breast cancer. Therefore, in some cases, tamoxifen may be replaced with the administration of a newer class of breast cancer drug called aromatase inhibitors, or AIs (Reynolds, 2007). The cost of AIs, however, can be as high as $18,000 for five years of treatment (Pollack, 2008). Some women are given AIs alone, and some receive them after the administration of tamoxifen (Goetz, Kamal, & Ames, 2008; Reynolds, 2007). In early clinical trials AIs outperformed tamoxifen, and there is evidence that AI are safer and far more tolerable than tamoxifen (National Cancer Institute, 2006). Certainly, patient comfort is a huge influence on quality of life and, in this and other instances, may justify the use of a newer drug even if efficacy is equivalent but not better.

One huge caveat is that not all new drugs are as effective as clinical trials first show them to be. This may be the case because new drugs have not been scrutinized in as many studies as older drugs that have been examined and reexamined through years of ongoing trails and retrospective studies. In the case of AIs, researchers are not yet sure whether new revelations about one or more genetic variations in breast cancer patients would have an impact on the drug's efficacy (Pollack, 2008). Research has emerged that the older, cheaper drug tamoxifen may be better suited for a subgroup of women who have genetic variations that successfully convert tamoxifen into endoxifen (Goetz et al., 2005; Lim, Desta, Flockhart, & Skaar, 2005; Stearns et al., 2003). Furthermore, it is the properties of endoxifen that fight certain breast cancer tumors (Goetz et al., 2005). For the majority of women with or recovering from hormone-receptor-positive breast cancer, this discovery may have little impact on their treatment going forward. Yet, for a subgroup, this information could influence the treatment and even the outcomes of their treatment.

Personalized medicine capitalizes on our growing knowledge of genetics and the pharmacogenetic interaction of a drug once it enters an individual's body (Buclin, Colombo, & Biollaz, 2008). Perhaps checking every breast cancer patient for the *CYP2D6* gene, the presence of which favors the metabolism of tamoxifen, could potentially lead to better outcomes through tailored care. However, the fact that a treatment algorithm is tailored to the patient does not imply that there might also be cost savings. This may be the case because as care becomes more tailored we may also see an increased need for specific training, or for visits with more specialists such as genetic counselors or other personnel needed to administer and interpret the tests. The field of personalized medicine is in its infancy, but it won't be for long; surely it will burgeon into a much larger industry calling for far more researchers, lab workers, and specialists (Pollack, 2008).

With the last couple of examples we want to make three points. First, newer drugs and new technology come with substantially higher costs. Even when we know that a cheaper treatment, test, or device may be just as effective as a more expensive alternative, patients may still demand and deserve the newer variety because of issues related to side effects and comfort. Second, even if we continue to use an older diagnostic test or treatment, the cost of care may still be inflationary due to advancing applications and follow-up care that are also related to quality-of-life issues. What we also know is that health conditions that were perhaps difficult to diagnose in past years may be treatable in the near future; however, this too comes with greater expenses. The advent of nanomedicine and the next wave of stents and artificial knees and hips, for example, promise improvements in well-being yet appear to offer only partial hope of lower costs to the patient, surgeon, and hospitals.

Finally, in this discussion we want to acknowledge the huge costs involved in bringing newer drugs, devices, and other treatments to market. "Newer" typically arrives only after a huge investment in terms of research and development. These costs reflect the spending on research and clinical trials, and the expense of bringing the drug to the consumer through marketing has sometimes mirrored or exceeded those initial investments (Kleyman, 2004). These costs are always on the rise, with more investment into more drugs driving spending. In the United States, pharmaceutical companies spent an estimated $58.8 billion in 2007 on developing and researching drugs (Pharmaceutical Research and Manufacturers of America [PhRMA], 2008). That figure marked a 43% increase from 2003 investment levels (AllBusiness, 2004), yet the number of medicines in development rose by only 25% in the same time period (PhRMA, 2008). A 2003 study found that the R&D costs for a single drug rose at an annual rate of about 7.4%, after the general inflation was taken into account (DiMasi, Hansen, & Grabowski, 2003).

2.4 HOW INCREASING HEALTH CARE COSTS IS A CAUSE OF CONFLICT

Certainly, there is a body of research that explores why U.S. public health spending far outpaces other OECD countries (Anderson & Frogner, 2008). The fast answer to this line of inquiry seems painfully simple: the whole package of drugs, devices, services, talent, and administration simply costs more in the United States than it does anywhere else (Anderson, Reinhardt, Hussey, & Petrosyan, 2003). This may seem like a rhetorical answer to a somewhat misplaced question. We could also say that the United States is one of the world's most populous developed nations, so of course our health expenditure is higher. But we must not forget that our health outcomes are worse, not better, than those of smaller nations. In truth this question looks at only part of the equation relating to costs; patient expectations in the United States, which are less easily quantified and understood, also play a major role in how we seek care and how it is delivered. We tackle this issue in the next chapter. But, before we move on to talk about expectations, let us look for a moment at an example of how inflationary costs influence the relationships among the stakeholders in the U.S. health care market.

Contentious standoffs between stakeholders result in rifts in trust and situations where everyone loses. For years now I have been preaching the return on investment of trust (Shore, 2005, 2007). When trust is absent, stakeholder conflict ensues, and this can lead to contentious standoffs that waste both money and time. One such stakeholder standoff occurred in early 2009, between Blue Cross Blue Shield of Massachusetts (BCBSMA) and Tufts Medical Center (Allen & Krasner, 2009). Tufts learned that BCBSMA was paying more per procedure to competing teaching hospitals, in particular Massachusetts General Hospital. Upon this discovery and without securing remediation, board members at Tufts Medical Center took the risky measure of announcing they would no longer accept the Blue Cross Blue Shield HMO because the insurer was not reimbursing the hospital adequately for care provided to patients. A company spokesperson for BCBSMA charged that Tufts Medical Center was "putting patients in the crossfire" by threatening to terminate coverage from the giant insurer while using brinkmanship to negotiate higher payments (Allen & Krasner). Tufts Medical Center's chief executive, Ellen Zane, countered that the hospital's doctors received up to 40% less than doctors at other area hospitals despite her hospital's high ranking for overall quality. She argued that Tufts is among the top three teaching hospitals in the state of Massachusetts and should receive reimbursements similar to those at the other top teaching hospitals (Allen & Krasner).

The resolution to this standoff, however, came only after trust was restored. Tufts Medical Center and BCBSMA agreed to very specific performance measures as a way to determine the cost of care. This went far beyond the pay-for-performance and quality measures that are used throughout the country, which ask rudimentary questions such as, "Did you give aspirin when cardiac patients came through the door?" Instead, Tufts agreed to be measured by specific quality standards as criteria for receiving higher payments (Allen & Krasner, 2009). We know that similar situations between providers and insurers are often just as contentious, and not as easily resolved. There are regions and states in the United States where a single provider may inhabit a dominant role and secure far higher reimbursements from insurers than do other, smaller providers. Conversely, there are areas where a single insurance giant is dominant and able to call the shots. In Chapter 5 we introduce a case study that looks at the very intricate issue of negotiating reimbursements from the perspective of various stakeholders.

The positive takeaway from the confrontation and subsequent resolution between Tufts and BCBSMA is that stakeholders *can* align their interests. But this begs the question of how we may better find places in the health care world where interests can be aligned before conflict occurs. We also must ask: can this type of stakeholder coordination happen more frequently, without contentious, money-wasting disruptions? These are the questions we address in coming chapters. One important analogy that serves us well when coordinating interest between stakeholders is the story of the Gordian knot.

2.5 THE GORDIAN KNOT AND THE PUSH-PULL DYNAMICS OF HEALTH CARE COSTS

The story of the Gordian knot dates back to ancient times when Alexander the Great was challenged to untie a trick knot. He soon found that pulling on one of the four threads dangling from the knot only tightened the tangle of rope. Rebuffed and frustrated by this problem, Alexander sliced through the knot with his sword (in other accounts he figures out a way to untie it). For some, the story serves as a metaphor for overcoming a problem by starting anew. For others, Alexander's move of cutting the knot is swift and decisive, but ultimately destructive. What use are a few broken pieces of twine, one might ask. Other questions follow: Is there a one-stroke

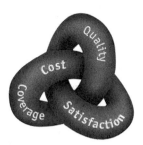

FIGURE 2.5 The Gordian knot.

solution to improving the value in U.S. health care? Can some stakeholders cut others out of the solution? The answer to these questions is a most definite no. The Gordian knot analogy serves to remind us that we can analyze the push–pull dynamics in the system. Figure 2.5 identifies the four core variables: cost, quality, coverage, and stakeholder satisfaction.

Often, but not always, losses and gains in the health care environment are seen in terms of cost and coverage to care, but as we mentioned earlier, this is an oversimplification. Higher costs can limit access to care, but as we see from the examples mentioned in this chapter, we need to consider not only access but also appropriate health care delivery. Limiting coverage for primary care and preventive services may actually drive up the delivery costs for health care in the long run, both for the patient and for other stakeholders. So here we begin to see how the stakeholders are intimately knotted together. If we pick up the knot and study it, we can soon see that for any given situation, additional variables will inevitably reveal themselves. Importantly, the four factors are critical variables that concern all stakeholders in health care. It is these factors that set expectations about health care delivery. A discussion of these factors may be seen as a kind of litmus test for health care stakeholders trying to seek alignment on any issue, big or small. Clearly, the Health Care and Education Reconciliation Act of 2010 was passed in an attempt to tackle these variables. In Chapter 3 we take a closer look at the nuances of some major cost- and coverage-limiting forces that play into the stakeholders' perception of health care delivery and how these perceptions influence expectations.

REFERENCES

Aaron, H. J. (2003). The costs of health care administration in the United States and Canada—questionable answers to a questionable question. *New England Journal of Medicine, 349*(8), 801–803.

AllBusiness. (2004, March 1). *Pharma R&D stats released.* Retrieved November 22, 2010, from http://www.allbusiness.com/company-activities-management/research-development/8256862-1.html

Allen, S. and J. Krasner (2009, January 6). Tufts to break with Blue Cross: Hospitals take high-risk step over doctor pay. *Boston Globe*, p. A1.

America's Health Insurance Plans. (2008, December 9). *Consumers and employers paying almost $90 billion due to under-payments to hospitals and physicians by Medicare and*

Medicaid. Retrieved November 22, 2010, from http://www.ahip.org/content/press release.aspx?docid=25218

Anderson, G. F., & Frogner, B. K. (2008). Health spending in OECD countries: Obtaining value per dollar. *Health Affairs (Millwood), 27*(6), 1718–1727.

Anderson, G. F., Reinhardt, U. E., Hussey, P. S., & Petrosyan, V. (2003). It's the prices, stupid: Why the United States is so different from other countries. *Health Affairs (Millwood), 22*(3), 89–105.

Begley, C. E., Vojvodic, R. W., Seo, M., & Burau, K. (2006). Emergency room use and access to primary care: Evidence from Houston, Texas. *Journal of Health Care for the Poor and Underserved, 17*(3), 610–624.

Brenner, D. J., & Hall, E. J. (2007). Computed tomography—an increasing source of radiation exposure. *New England Journal of Medicine, 357*(22), 2277–2284.

Buclin, T., Colombo, S., & Biollaz, J. (2008). [Pharmacogenetic testing: Soon before every prescription?]. *Revue Medicale de la Suisse Romande, 4*(165), 1666–1670.

Casalino, L. P., Nicholson, S., Gans, D. N., Hammons, T., Morra, D., Karrison, T., et al. (2009). What does it cost physician practices to interact with health insurance plans? *Health Affairs (Millwood), 28*(4), w533–w543.

Cavazos Galvan, M. (2006). Asthma in emergency department. *Guidelines, physicians and patients. Revista Alergia Mexico, 53*(4), 136–143.

Centers for Disease Control and Prevention. (2007). *The state of aging and health in America 2007 report*. Retrieved March 26, 2009, from the Centers for Disease Control and Prevention Web site, http://www.cdc.gov/aging/saha.htm

Centers for Medicare and Medicaid Services. (2005). *Medicaid program—general information*. Retrieved November 22, 2010, from the Centers for Medicare and Medicaid Services Web site, http://www.cms.gov/MedicaidGenInfo/

Chernew, M., Cutler, D. M., & Keenan, P. S. (2005). Increasing health insurance costs and the decline in insurance coverage. *Health Services Research, 40*(4), 1021–1039.

Cohen, R. A., Martinez, M. E., & Ward BW. (2010). *Health insurance coverage: Early release of estimates from the National Health Interview Survey, 2009* [Electronic version]. Retrieved July 15, 2010, from the Centers for Disease Control and Prevention Web site, http://www.cdc.gov/nchs/data/nhis/earlyrelease/insur201006.htm

Colamery, S. N. (2003). *Medicare: Current issues and background*. Hauppauge, NY: Nova Science Publishers, Inc.

DiMasi, J. A., Hansen, R. W., & Grabowski, H. G. (2003). The price of innovation: New estimates of drug development costs. *Journal of Health Economics, 22*(2), 151–185.

Dobson, A., Davanzo, J., & Sen, N. (2006). The cost-shift payment "hydraulic": Foundation, history, and implications. *Health Affairs (Millwood), 25*(1), 22–33.

Edlund, B. J., Lufkin, S. R., & Franklin, B. (2003). Long-term care planning for baby boomers: Addressing an uncertain future. *Online Journal of Issues in Nursing, 8*(2), 3. Retrieved November 22, 2010, from http://www.nursingworld.org/MainMenuCategories/ANA Marketplace/ANAPeriodicals/OJIN/TableofContents/Volume82003/No2May2003/ CarePlanningforBabyBoomers.aspx

Finkelstein, E. A., Fiebelkorn, I. C., & Wang, G. (2003). National medical spending attributable to overweight and obesity: How much, and who's paying? *Health Affairs (Millwood), Web Exclusives*, w219–w226.

Finkelstein, E. A., Trogdon, J. G., Cohen, J. W., & Dietz, W. (2009). Annual medical spending attributable to obesity: Payer- and service-specific estimates. *Health Affairs (Millwood), 28*(5), w822–w831.

Fox, W., & Pickering, J. (2008). *Hospital and physician cost shift: Payment level comparison of Medicare, Medicaid, and commercial payers*. Seattle, WA: Milliman; 2008. Retrieved November 23, 2010, from http://www.cbia.com/ieb/ag/CostOfCare/RisingCosts/Milliman_HospitalPhysicianCostShift12_08.pdf

Franco Sassi, M. D., Cecchini, M., & Rusticelli, E. (2009). *The obesity epidemic: Analysis of past and projected future trends in selected OECD countries*. Paris: Organisation for Economic Co-operation and Development.

Goetz, M. P., Kamal, A., & Ames, M. M. (2008). Tamoxifen pharmacogenomics: The role of CYP2D6 as a predictor of drug response. *Clinical Pharmacology & Therapeutics, 83*(1), 160–166.

Goetz, M. P., Rae, J. M., Suman, V. J., Safgren, S. L., Ames, M. M., Visscher, D. W., et al. (2005). Pharmacogenetics of tamoxifen biotransformation is associated with clinical outcomes of efficacy and hot flashes. *Journal of Clinical Oncology, 23*(36), 9312–9318.

Hall, A. G., Harman, J. S., & Zhang, J. (2008). Lapses in Medicaid coverage: Impact on cost and utilization among individuals with diabetes enrolled in Medicaid. *Medical Care, 46*(12), 1219–1225.

Hall, A. G., Lemak, C. H., Steingraber, H., & Schaffer, S. (2008). Expanding the definition of access: It isn't just about health insurance. *Journal of Health Care for the Poor and Underserved, 19*(2), 625–638.

Himmelstein, D. U., & Woolhandler, S. (1986). Cost without benefit. Administrative waste in U.S. health care. *New England Journal of Medicine, 314*(7), 441–445.

Himmelstein, D. U., & Woolhandler, S. (1989). A national health program for the United States. A physicians' proposal. *New England Journal of Medicine, 320*(2), 102–108.

Himmelstein, D. U., & Woolhandler, S. (1993). The American health care system—Medicare. *New England Journal of Medicine, 328*(24), 1789; author reply 1790.

Hoot, N. R. and D. Aronsky (2008). Systematic review of emergency department crowding: causes, effects, and solutions. *Annals of Emergency Medicine, 52*(2), 126–136.

InSight Health Corp. (2009). *What is an open MRI?* Retrieved August 7, 2009, from http://www.insighthealth.com/services.asp?mid=2

Jamison, D. T., & Sandbu, M. E. (2001). Global health. WHO ranking of health system performance. *Science, 293*(5535), 1595–1596.

Janney, M. (2007, October 1). Open MRI alleviates problems: WVU will put new machine to use soon. *Dominion Post*, pp. 9a–11a.

Keehan, S., Sisko, A., Truffer, C., Smith, S., Cowan, C., Poisal, J., et al. (2008). Health spending projections through 2017: The baby-boom generation is coming to Medicare. *Health Affairs (Millwood), 27*(2), w145–w155.

Kellermann, A. L. (2006). Crisis in the emergency department. *New England Journal of Medicine, 355*(13), 1300–1303.

Kleyman, P. (2004). The truth about the critical condition of overdosed America. *Aging Today, 25*(6). Retrieved November 22, 2010, from http://www.asaging.org/publications/dbase/AT/AT-256-The_Truth_About.pdf

Lim, Y. C., Desta, Z., Flockhart, D. A., & Skaar, T. C. (2005). Endoxifen (4-hydroxy-N-desmethyl-tamoxifen) has anti-estrogenic effects in breast cancer cells with potency similar to 4-hydroxy-tamoxifen. *Cancer Chemotherapy and Pharmacology, 55*(5), 471–478.

Luft, H. S., Garnick, D. W., Hughes, R. G., Hunt, S. S., McPhee, S. J., & Robinson, J. C. (1988). Hospital competition, cost, and medical practice. *Journal of Medical Practice Management, 4*(1), 10–15.

Manhattan Institute for Policy Research. (2007). *Talking points with the author: Regina Herzlinger*. Retrieved October 9, 2009, from http://www.manhattan-institute.org/health care/talking_points.htm

Martin, P. P., & Weaver, D. A. (2005). Social security: A program and policy history. *Social Security Bulletin, 66*(1), 1–15.

Mendelson, D., & Carino, T. V. (2005). Evidence-based medicine in the United States—de rigueur or dream deferred? *Health Affairs (Millwood), 24*(1), 133–136.

Mitchell, J. M. (2008). Utilization trends for advanced imaging procedures: Evidence from individuals with private insurance coverage in California. *Medical Care, 46*(5), 460–466.

Moorman, J. E., Rudd, R. A., Johnson, C. A., King, M., Minor, P., Bailey, C., et al. (2007). National surveillance for asthma—United States, 1980–2004. *Morbidity and Mortality Weekly Report, 56*(SS08), 18–54.

National Cancer Institute. (2006, October 20). *Advanced breast cancer patients benefit more from aromatase inhibitors than tamoxifen*. Retrieved March 27, 2009, from the National Cancer Institute Web site, http://www.cancer.gov/clinicaltrials/results/aromatase-inhibitors1006

Newton, M. F., Keirns, C. C., Cunningham, R., Hayward, R. A., & Stanley, R. (2008). Uninsured adults presenting to U.S. emergency departments: Assumptions vs. data. *Journal of the American Medical Association, 300*(16), 1914–1924.

Nolte, E., & McKee, C. M. (2008). Measuring the health of nations: Updating an earlier analysis. *Health Affairs (Millwood), 27*(1), 58–71.

Organisation for Economic Co-operation and Development. (2010). *OECD health data 2010*. Available from the Organisation for Economic Co-operation and Development Web site, http://www.oecd.org/document/30/0,3343,en_2649_34631_12968734_1_1_1_1,00.html

Peppe, E. M., Mays, J. W., Chang, H. C., Becker, E., & DiJulio, B. (2007). *Characteristics of frequent emergency department users*. Menlo Park, CA: The Henry J. Kaiser Family Foundation.

Pharmaceutical Research and Manufacturers of America. (2008). *R&D Spending by U.S. Biopharmaceutical Companies Reaches Record $58.8 Billion in 2007* [Press release]. Washington, DC: Pharmaceutical Research and Manufacturers of America.

Pham, J. C., R. Patel, et al. (2006). The effects of ambulance diversion: a comprehensive review. *Academic Emergency Medicine, 13*(11), 1220–1227.

Pollack, A. (2008, December 30). Patient's DNA may be signal to tailor medication. *New York Times*, p. A1.

Reynolds, S. (2007). Aromatase inhibitors come of age [Electronic version]. *NCI Cancer Bulletin: Eliminating the Suffering and Death Due to Cancer, 4*, 5–6. Retrieved October 6, 2009, from the National Cancer Institute Web site, http://www.cancer.gov/ncicancer bulletin/NCI_Cancer_Bulletin_030607.pdf

Roduit, C., S. Scholtens, et al. (2009). Asthma at 8 years of age in children born by caesarean section. *Thorax, 64*(2), 107–113.

Sack, K., & Zezima, K. (2009, January 22). Growing need for Medicaid strains states. *New York Times*, p. A25.

Schoen, C., Osborn, R., How, S. K., Doty, M. M., & Peugh, J. (2009). In chronic condition: Experiences of patients with complex health care needs, in eight countries, 2008. *Health Affairs (Millwood), 28*(1), w1–w16.

Shore, D. A. (2005). *The trust prescription for healthcare: Building your reputation with consumers*. Chicago, IL: Health Administration Press.

Shore, D. A. (Ed.). (2007). *The trust crisis in healthcare: Causes, consequences, and cures* (1st ed.). New York, NY: Oxford University Press.

Smith-Bindman, R., Miglioretti, D. L., & Larson, E. B. (2008). Rising use of diagnostic medical imaging in a large integrated health system. *Health Affairs (Millwood), 27*(6), 1491–1502.

Spellman, L. (2008). Lack of primary care doctors presents a major challenge. *UNMC Today*. Retrieved November 23, 2010, from the University of Nebraska Medical Center Web site, http://app1.unmc.edu/publicaffairs/todaysite/sitefiles/today_full.cfm?match=5169

Spivey, M., & Kellermann, A. L. (2009). Rescuing the safety net. *New England Journal of Medicine, 360*(25), 2598–2601.

Stearns, V., Johnson, M. D., Rae, J. M., Morocho, A., Novielli, A., Bhargava, P., et al. (2003). Active tamoxifen metabolite plasma concentrations after coadministration of tamoxifen and the selective serotonin reuptake inhibitor paroxetine. *Journal of the National Cancer Institute, 95*(23), 1758–1764.

Studdert, D. M., Mello, M. M., Sage, W. M., DesRoches, C. M., Peugh, J., Zapert, K., et al. (2005). Defensive medicine among high-risk specialist physicians in a volatile malpractice environment. *Journal of the American Medical Association, 293*(21), 2609–2617.

Thomson Reuters Healthcare. (2009, June 22). *Thomson Reuters study finds Baby Boomers and Generation X face healthcare cost hurdles.* Retrieved November 23, 2010, from http://thomsonreuters.com/content/press_room/healthcare/tr_study_finds_baby_boomers_genx

U.S. Government Accountability Office. (2008). *Medicare part B imaging services: Rapid spending growth and shift to physician offices indicate need for CMS to consider additional management practices* (No. GAO-08-452). Washington, DC: U.S. Government Accountability Office.

Weber, E. J., J. A. Showstack, et al. (2008). Are the uninsured responsible for the increase in emergency department visits in the United States? *Annals of Emergency Medicine, 52*(2), 108–115.

Woolhandler, S., Campbell, T., & Himmelstein, D. U. (2003). Costs of health care administration in the United States and Canada. *New England Journal of Medicine, 349*(8), 768–775.

Woolhandler, S., Campbell, T., & Himmelstein, D. U. (2004). Health care administration in the United States and Canada: Micromanagement, macro costs. *International Journal of Health Services, 34*(1), 65–78.

Woolhandler, S., & Himmelstein, D. U. (1991). The deteriorating administrative efficiency of the U.S. health care system. *New England Journal of Medicine, 324*(18), 1253–1258.

Woolhandler, S., & Himmelstein, D. U. (1994). Correction: The deteriorating administrative efficiency of the U.S. health care system. *New England Journal of Medicine, 331*(5), 336.

Woolhandler, S., & Himmelstein, D. U. (1995). Extreme risk—the new corporate proposition for physicians. *New England Journal of Medicine, 333*(25), 1706–1708.

Woolhandler, S., & Himmelstein, D. U. (1997). Costs of care and administration at for-profit and other hospitals in the United States. *New England Journal of Medicine, 336*(11), 769–774.

Woolhandler, S., & Himmelstein, D. U. (1999). When money is the mission—the high costs of investor-owned care. *New England Journal of Medicine, 341*(6), 444–446.

Woolhandler, S., Himmelstein, D. U., & Lewontin, J. P. (1993). Administrative costs in U.S. hospitals. *New England Journal of Medicine, 329*(6), 400–403.

World Health Organization. (2000). Annex Table 10: Health systems performance in all member states, WHO indexes, estimates for 1997. In World Health Organization,

The world health report 2000: Health systems: Improving performance. Geneva, Switzerland: World Health Organization.

World Health Organization. (2008). *Mortality and burden of disease* [Data file]. Retrieved February 17, 2009, from the World Health Organization Web site, http://www.who.int/whosis/whostat/1.xls

World Health Organization. (2009). *Obesity.* Retrieved March 30, 2009, from http://www.who.int/topics/obesity/en/

Wright, R. J. (2006). Health effects of socially toxic neighborhoods: The violence and urban asthma paradigm. *Clinics in Chest Medicine, 27*(3), 413–421.

Wu, P., W. D. Dupont, et al. (2008). Evidence of a causal role of winter virus infection during infancy in early childhood asthma. *American Journal of Respiratory and Critical Care Medicine, 178*(11), 1123–1129.

3 Our Great Expectations

3.1 THE VIAGRA EFFECT: SOCIETAL EXPECTATIONS ABOUT GOOD HEALTH

Here we detangle the issue of the rising cost of health care from things that are harder to measure, such as our expectations about the level of health care we need and deserve. When I discuss expectation in the classroom, I find that many graduate students and executive education participants quickly enter into debates over health care policy and the government's role in crafting new reforms—but we are not addressing policy in this book. We will identify, however, how expectations play a major role in the push–pull between the stakeholder groups. This chapter looks at how and where expectations of different stakeholder groups diverge. We frequently hear that medicine in the United States is the best in the world. Yet we know that our health outcomes, on aggregate, put us far behind the top performers in our peer group. We have wonderful technologies and hospitals staffed with a wide variety of highly skilled professionals. We have an elaborate network of specialists, many of whom may be among the most reputable in their field. But another huge caveat is that we also have very low levels of satisfaction, among patients and doctors alike.

Often when we talk about our health care expectations and how health care is delivered, we encounter a question couched in these terms: is health care a human right, or a responsibility? We encounter health care stakeholders on both sides of this debate. We have those insisting that health care is a basic human right, just as a fair trial is designated as a basic right. We find others who believe it is a responsibility, to be taken up by a number of stakeholders, such as employers, the government, and the patient himself or herself. We have others still who would rather not reveal their hand. Two very well argued perspectives appearing in the *British Medical Journal* show how the debate on health care as a human right can go either way (Barlow, 1999; Berwick, Davidoff, Hiatt, & Smith, 2001; Berwick, Hiatt, Janeway, & Smith, 1997; Smith, Hiatt, & Berwick, 1999).

One perspective argues that health care is difficult to define, and that what constitutes health care is unclear. It asks whether making a list of basic necessities within health care is too difficult. For example, if you compare treatments like organ transplant, infertility treatment, and cosmetic surgery, who decides what is a basic necessity and what is not (Barlow, 1999)? The opposing perspective argues that health care is an undeniable human right, yet even those arguing this point do not offer a clear definition of what health care encompasses, or how it should be delivered. As we mention in Chapter 2, and will repeat here, where you stand depends on where you sit. This means that each stakeholder comes to the table with a unique perspective that is influenced by how, when, and where the individual was trained; whom he or she works for; or what industry or group the stakeholder is representing. In the United States, some stakeholders might see health care as a human right, while others might instead believe that employers have a right to attract skilled labor by offering a good health-benefits package as part of work compensation.

The Tavistock group, a committee of concerned academics from different stakeholder groups and countries, set out to define a shared moral framework within the world of health care (Berwick, Davidoff, et al., 2001; Berwick, Hiatt, et al., 1997; Smith et al., 1999). They first met more than ten years ago because of a mutual concern over the sustainability of health care delivery. This group included participants from the United States, United Kingdom, Mexico, and South Africa. They banded together because they felt a need to "bring all stakeholders in health care into a more consistent moral framework." The reasoning behind this effort was that the increasing rate of health care consumption and expectations would eventually limit resources and curtail quality delivery—a notion akin to Hardin's tragedy of the commons (Hardin, 1968). They were also concerned that the squeeze on health care delivery would lead to falling health outcomes. The group was also a strong advocate of health care as a basic human right (Berwick, Davidoff, et al., 2001; Berwick, Hiatt, et al., 1997; Smith et al., 1999).

In their investigations, the Tavistock group hit on one very important trend. From a sociological and cultural perspective, there is a greater taste for health services right now than ever before. This means that we are more willing to seek treatments for problems that one generation ago were considered to be simply part of aging. Here is a classic example: It used to be that when we hit our golden years we were not to expect a healthy and fulfilling sex life. But now, with a choice of safe and effective impotency drugs that may be covered by a number of private health insurance providers, erectile dysfunction is treatable (Keith, 2000). Delicately put, a retired couple can now believe that sex is an attainable part of their life. One generation ago, this demographic may have not expected to still be having sex into their twilight years. Undoubtedly, aging Americans expect to do more and to feel better in their retirement than previous generations did. It used to be that if you reached 80, you did not expect to be hitting the golf course or the swimming pool. However, with knee and hip replacements becoming routine and safe, America's teeming retirement communities are full of just such active retirees.

Expectations are a difficult thing to measure empirically and, by extension, are also difficult to align. Expectations about good health and treatment are notions that are set, in part, by the various types of providers, insurers, employers, drug companies, news media, researchers, government, friends, and family. The list goes on, of course, as any individual may be influenced by any number of information sources and people. To illustrate this, we go back to our example from Chapter 2 about breast cancer and the new revelations about tamoxifen. In this example, we want to show just how many stakeholders are involved in setting health expectations.

The *New York Times* article mentioned in Chapter 2 describes a breast cancer patient, Jody Uslan (Pollack, 2008). She, like an increasing number of breast cancer patients, had taken the newly available genetic test to determine whether her body was able to transform tamoxifen to endoxifen. The host's ability to transform the drug from tamoxifen to endoxifen is believed to be a key step needed to fight a possible return of certain breast cancers (Higgins & Stearns, 2009). But following the genetic test, Uslan was told she did not have the genes believed necessary to metabolize tamoxifen into the cancer-fighting endoxifen. Ms. Uslan described feeling "devastated" after learning that the tamoxifen she had been taking was not helping her prevent a return of cancer (Pollack, 2008).

Some researchers have now begun to speak out against routine genetic testing for breast cancer patients like Ms. Uslan. As recently as 2009, a group of scientists recommended that patients forgo genetic tests that determine whether an individual has the *CYP2D6* genotype (Higgins, Rae, Flockhart, Hayes, & Stearns, 2009). In a leading medical journal, Dr. Michaela J. Higgins and colleagues (2009) wrote that because the revelations were gleaned from data gathered from prospective studies, the recent findings were not robust enough to change or even modify clinical guidelines on the use of tamoxifen just yet. These scientists reasoned that more work was necessary to confirm and investigate the hypothesis about tamoxifen metabolism. The scientists' argument is a logical one. However, imagine for a moment that you are a breast cancer patient who has read the article in the *New York Times* about personalized medicine and the use of tamoxifen (Pollack, 2008). No doubt, you might still ask for the genetic test from your doctor or at the clinic where you receive treatment. Chances are you would probably want to find out whether a drug is likely to be effective or not, even as the meaning of the revelations is still being investigated.

This example highlights the unique role that a number of stakeholder groups play in health expectations here in the United States. How many stakeholders appear in this scenario? There are the patient, the hospitals, the doctors, the researchers, and the news media. Look closer at this example and you will see how many more stakeholders are intimately knotted into the issue of setting expectations. We have the biotechnology company that has developed the genetic test. We will probably have lab technicians and genetics counselors who will offer interpretations and advice about the tests' outcomes. As we went to press, the U.S. Food and Drug Administration (FDA) was getting tough on companies that market and sell genetic tests (Pollack, 2010). Previously, these tests, unlike drugs and most devices, could be marketed without FDA approval. This will change, however, as the FDA is beginning to insist on things such as a mention of gene–drug interactions on the labels of a handful of medicines (Pollack, 2008, 2010). So we also have regulators who may be increasingly interested in controlling users' expectations surrounding results from genetic tests. We also probably have an insurer, and possibly an employer, or the government (in the case of government-sponsored programs like Medicare and Medicaid), who, although not mentioned in the above story, are likely to be playing a role in decision making about treatment reimbursements.

In this brief example, we may have clinicians who, to a certain extent, are under pressure to please their patients, who are also their customers. Patients, who are increasingly armed with medical information, may challenge or switch providers if they feel expectations are not being met. This means we have more than one provider competing for the breast cancer patient, and possibly a private payer that may not cover the cost of a genetic test as routine breast cancer care. The payer may be an employer who has designed the benefits package as part of overall compensation, maybe after receiving advice from an outside health consultant. The treatment may be carried out inside a hospital that bases its charges on a per diem system or on inpatient and outpatient charges. Some of the price points for these rates may have been influenced by the government, depending on the region. Some patients may be reliant not on employee-based insurance, but on insurance through the federal programs.

Also holding stakes in this particular situation are cancer support groups, cancer institutes, and local or national breast cancer coalitions and foundations. All of these special-interest groups may be setting expectations on a particular aspect of care. Indeed, in order to appreciate the paradox behind rising cost and the patients' rising health expectations, we must appreciate the vast diversity of our stakeholder groups and how they influence expectations.

3.2 THE FLIP SIDE TO THE VIAGRA EFFECT: DIMINISHING HEALTH CARE ACCESS AND EXPECTATIONS

We have considered rising expectations and the notion of wellness. As it turns out, for many millions of people residing in the United States, falling expectations have become the norm. It is hard to track exactly where this trend began. Falling expectations due to lack of health insurance coverage and an inability to afford doctor visits, drugs, or care did not start with the current tough economic times. A Centers for Disease Control and Prevention (CDC) survey estimated that at least 46.3 million people living in the United States are considered to be nonelderly uninsured persons (Cohen, 2010). Approximately 75 million adults experience a period with either no insurance or underinsurance over the course of a year (The Commonwealth Fund Commission on a High Performance Health System, 2008; Glied & Mahato, 2008; U.S. Census Bureau, 2007). For many working-age adults, the trend of not

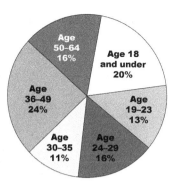

FIGURE 3.1 Breakdown of uninsurance by age. From "Analysis of the March 2008 Current Population Survey" by S. Glied & B. Mahato, 2008, The Commonwealth Fund. Retrieved January 5, 2011, from http://www.commonwealthfund.org/~/media/Files/Publications/Testimony/2009/Apr/Testimony%20Young%20and%20Vulnerable/PPT%20and%20PDF/PDF%20City%20Council%20Hearing%204%2023%2009%20Figures%20FINAL.pdf Adapted with permission from the Commonwealth Fund.

having insurance, or of being underinsured, has persisted and even worsened for more than a decade (Ahluwalia & Bolen, 2008; Cohen, 2010; Himmelstein, Woolhandler, & Wolfe, 1992; U.S. Census Bureau, 2007). This is especially true for the U.S. youth who are transitioning from school age to working-age adults (Collins & Nicholson, 2010). To see a breakdown of uninsurance by age, please refer to Figure 3.1; also see Figure 3.2, which details periods of uninsurance in the youth populations (Glied & Mahato, 2008; Collins & Nicholson, 2010).

After looking at the figures on under- and uninsurance, it may not be surprising to learn that an estimated 29 million Americans have debts related to medical expenses (Seifert & Rukavina, 2006), and anywhere between 17% and 55% of bankruptcies in America may attribute their financial slide to unpaid medical expenses (Dranove & Millenson, 2006; Himmelstein, Warren, Thorne, & Woolhandler, 2005).

A great number of people in the United States may have excellent health care coverage, perhaps funding it through a tailored employer-linked benefits package, as well as personal finances. It almost goes without saying that those who do not have good health care coverage due to lack of insurance, underinsurance, and limited resources still desire thorough health care. But how are these high expectations met? Many would argue that these high expectations eventually translate into poor satisfaction with the delivery of care. In the worst-case scenario, getting health care has not just cost patients their satisfaction; it has also led them to financial ruin. This is a phenomenon that some have termed "medical bankruptcy." Academics disagree as to the extent that medical expenses contribute to personal bankruptcy in the United States, with estimates falling between 17% and 55% (Dranove & Millenson, 2006; Himmelstein, Warren, et al., 2005; Seifert & Rukavina, 2006).

Someone once put it to me as an analogy (and I am paraphrasing here): getting health care in the United States is sort of like the guy who offers you a ride to work in his Mercedes. When you have the offer, you can coast along in the comfort and security of a luxury car. But when he leaves without you, you are pretty much on your own. Perhaps you take your chances by walking a great distance without an

Time spent without insurance

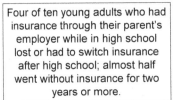
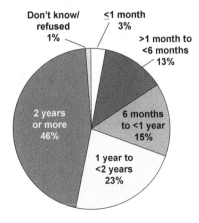

FIGURE 3.2 What to expect as a youth in the United States. Adapted from *Rite of Passage: Young Adults and the Affordable Care Act of 2010* [Issue brief], by.Collins, S. R., & Nicholson, J. L. (2010). The Commonwealth Fund, http://www.commonwealthfund.org/~/media/Files/Publications/Issue%20Brief/2010/May/1404_Collins_rite_of_passage_2010_v3.pdf; also see *The Commonwealth Fund Survey of Young Adults* (2009). Adapted with permission from the Commonwealth Fund.

umbrella—but you may get caught in bad weather. Or, maybe you decide to splurge on a cab ride every now and again. You do this because you have no car and there is no alternate transportation to get you where you need to go. Nowhere is someone saying, "Hey, driving that Mercedes is just one way to travel; you may also want to use this rapid transport system, which is just as safe and reliable but much more affordable."

In response to this health professional's analogy, I reminded her that there is an elaborate safety-net system to deliver health care to those who do not get coverage through employment. Many millions of people do get treatment and access to excellent health care through publicly funded coverage like Medicaid, Medicare, the Children's Health Insurance Program, or military and veteran health care. For those who are not eligible for these programs, there are free clinics provided by hundreds of safety-net hospitals. Despite my response, the analogy struck a cord with others, and soon they were agreeing that, indeed, for many residents in the United States, there is a sense of being left out of health care altogether. Just in contemplating the medical bankruptcy figures, even the lower estimates alone would lead most to conclude that many Americans might believe there are few alternatives when faced with a health problem: one meets with either financial disaster or the consequences of a lack of treatment.

As was outlined in previous chapters, the safety-net system has also deteriorated somewhat. As hospitals face increases in the costs of care delivery, they may find they have no choice but to shut down or consolidate free clinics. These problems have caught the media's attention in recent years, and stories about struggling public hospital clinics abound (Sack & Zezima, 2009). Nevertheless, it is important to note that the U.S. government does support one of the largest publicly funded systems of health care coverage in the world in terms of pure numbers (DeNavas-Walt, Proctor, & Smith, 2008). By 2008 estimates, there were approximately 87.4 million people covered by government-funded health insurance. The number of people in the United States relying on publicly funded coverage is greater than the population of the United Kingdom, Canada, or Australia—all countries that provide universal public health care. Additionally, those who are uninsured often rely on care provided by hospital emergency departments and/or free clinics at safety-net hospitals scattered across the country. When we went to press, the Health Care and Education Reconciliation Act of 2010 had been adopted not long ago. No doubt, the numbers of uninsured patients will likely change substantially in years to come; but many issues about coordination, quality, cost, and delivery of care will remain front and center.

Perhaps more accurately, the health care professional's analogy was about a growing dissatisfaction with the delivery of care. A survey conducted back in 2001 indicated that Medicare patients were, on average, more satisfied with their coverage than those who have private insurance (Davis, Schoen, Doty, & Tenney, 2002). This is despite the fact that it is commonly seen as far more preferable to have private health insurance. However, the same survey also noted that Medicare beneficiaries with no outpatient prescription drug coverage were far more likely to have problems filling their prescriptions (Davis et al.). This highlights the fact that people without medical insurance, people with limited insurance, or even those who are fully covered but lack a prescription drug benefit have always been in a particularly precarious position. They may remain uninsured because they do not qualify for public insurance. Instead, they may be avoiding or delaying care, and even skipping their prescribed drugs, for fear of the additional expenses. Yet, as we saw in Chapter 2, avoiding basic care may lead to higher expenses in urgent treatment down the road (Hall, Harman, & Zhang, 2008; Hall, Lemak, Steingraber, & Schaffer, 2008).

When we went to press, opting out of treatment had been and continued to be a growing trend. One example points to a steep increase in prescription abandonment (Wolters Kluwer Health, 2009). This happens when patients fill their prescriptions at a pharmacy but fail to collect them, perhaps because they cannot afford them. Evidence points to a spike in this behavior as the economy began to fail in 2008 (Wolters Kluwer Health, 2009). Indeed, while this example is telling, there is plenty of evidence that expectations began to fall long before the economy took a nosedive. Falling expectations may be linked to increasing health disparities due, in part, to trends of lost of coverage, price increases, and poor delivery, which causes diminishing health care coordination (Ahluwalia & Bolen, 2008). The number of people with full health insurance has always varied, in part because of states like Massachusetts that have implemented universal coverage, or other states that have been trying to increase Medicaid coverage (U.S. Census Bureau, 2007).

In downturns, we see the number of uninsured people increase because employer-based health insurance is proportional to how the economy is performing (U.S. Census Bureau, 2007). As the economy worsens or companies feel that pinch, they drop coverage, or they might pass along the comparatively higher cost to the employee in the form of higher premiums or higher deductibles (Chernew, Cutler, & Keenan, 2005). An individual without insurance falls into the state commonly referred to as "uninsured," but many individuals face a gray area of "underinsurance"—having some coverage or being intermittently insured. When comparing our residents with those of other countries, the United States has a much larger proportion of people who do not get care because of cost or the fear of incurring costs (Commonwealth Fund, 2008). You can see the comparable percentages in Figure 3.3, which exhibits the more recent findings from the Commonwealth Fund National Scorecard on U.S. health system performance; older surveys show this trend is not new (Schoen & Osborn, 2004).

If workers are laid off, or if they need to switch jobs or change from full time to part time, for example, they may suddenly not be able to afford health insurance for some portion of a year. Typically this situation results in periods where the workers and their family members face breaks in health coverage that can contribute to poorer health outcomes or less than ideal access to care (Leininger, 2009; Lenzer, 2008; Oswald, Bodurtha, Willis, & Moore, 2007). This phenomenon is commonly referred to as *churning* (Klein, Glied, & Ferry, 2005; Saunders & Alexander, 2009). Those who qualify for government-sponsored insurance may be in a slightly better position to access services than those who recently had private insurance but have lost their coverage. This is a central issue that the Health Care and Education

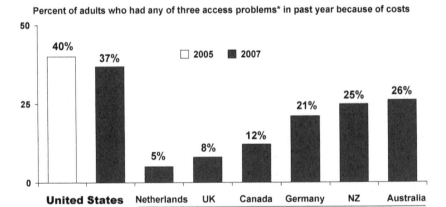

FIGURE 3.3 An international comparison of access problems.
*The Commonwealth Fund Health Survey looks at three access problems: (1) did not get medical care because of cost of doctor's visit; (2) skipped medical test, treatment, or follow-up because of cost; and (3) did not fill prescription or skipped doses because of cost. UK: United Kingdom; NZ: New Zealand. From *The Commonwealth Fund Commission on a High Performance Health System. (2008). Why not the best? Results from the national scorecard on U.S. health system performance, 2008* [Electronic version]. The Commonwealth Fund, http://www.commonwealthfund.org/Content/Publications/Fund-Reports/2008/Jul/Why-Not-the-Best-Results-from-the-National-Scorecard-on-U-S-Health-System-Performance-2008.aspx. Reproduced with permission from the Commonwealth Fund.

Reconciliation Act of 2010 was designed to address. However, populations that are traditionally dependent on government-sponsored health insurance have high rates of chronic illness and of nonadherence (Kennedy, Tuleu, & Mackay, 2008). Instances of rehospitalization among patients with Medicare are more frequent, longer, and more costly (Jencks, Williams, & Coleman, 2009). Health care coverage, or lack of it, is just part of the falling expectations; the other part of the equation is wrapped up in how care is delivered.

Another big problem that influences expectations, of insured and uninsured alike, is the chronic lack of patient coordination in health care delivery. This problem was first noted three decades ago (Cummins, Smith, & Inui, 1980). It has been blamed for increasing administrative costs, and it contributes to our dangerously high medical error rate (Moore, Wisnivesky, Williams, & McGinn, 2003). Problems in patient coordination may be related to a failure to relay information such as test results before hospital discharge (Roy et al., 2005). It can also come about due to a lack of communication between hospitals and primary care physicians and specialists (Kripalani et al., 2007). Yet it also may be traced back to staff and physician inability to correctly input data into the patients' records (O'Donnell et al., 2009). Commonwealth Fund survey reports show that the care-coordination gap is largest in the United States, compared to care coordination in other developed nations such as Australia and the United Kingdom (Schoen & Osborn, 2004). Figure 3.4 offers a comparison of the percentage of people agreeing with this statement across Australia, Canada, New Zealand, the United Kingdom, and the United States.

Even patients with employers that buy into the best possible insurance coverage may receive mediocre care due to poor patient coordination. It should come as no surprise, then, that at one end of the health care spectrum we see patients so frustrated or disillusioned that they are willing to pay a retainer to a physician for more thorough attention and coordination, a service often known as "concierge" or "boutique" care. So far, according to one estimate, only about a thousand doctors have changed to this concierge-care business model in the United States, but in doing so they have halved the number of patients they see while maintaining or

I have seen doctors in the past 2 years but:	AUS	CAN	NZ	UK	US
My test results or records were not available at time of appointment.	12	14	13	13	17
My doctor ordered tests that had already been done (duplication).	7	6	7	4	14
I received conflicting information from different doctors.	18	14	14	14	18
I experienced at least one of the above.	28	26	25	24	31

FIGURE 3.4 Care coordination. AUS: Australia; CAN: Canada; NZ: New Zealand; UK: United Kingdom; US: United States. Adapted from C. Schoen, & R. Osborn, R., 2004, *The Commonwealth Fund 2004 International Health Policy Survey of Primary Care in Five Countries.* Washington, DC: The Commonwealth Fund. Adapted with permission from the Commonwealth Fund.

increasing their revenues (Jenkins, 2008). Typically, concierge care allows you to access your physician 24/7. If you need to see a specialist, your doctor may accompany you to the appointment, records in hand. Often, he or she will discuss the treatment, diagnosis, and other details about your care with the specialist or a team of specialists, ensuring that you, as a priority patient, get a treatment plan that is individually tailored (Zuger, 2005).

Up until this point we have mainly touched on the patient's satisfaction with health care delivery. We will turn briefly to the doctors' satisfaction with the business of providing care. At the beginning of this chapter we discussed how patients have a greater taste for health care now than they did generations ago. In many ways their expectations for a higher standard of living have been boosted by a great number of medical breakthroughs and successful treatment regimes. A typical patient-consumer in the United States may be inclined to visit his or her physician after having read or heard an advertisement. The same may be true for individuals having visited informational, drug- and treatment-specific Web sites. In the meantime, the "informed" patient-consumer brings greater challenges, and opportunities, to physicians.

For example, doctors must guide increasingly demanding patients to appropriate care, and thwart litigious patients and the extra costs they bring. In certain circumstances doctors may provide care to a portion of patients whose reimbursements are below the cost of care (as is the case with Medicaid patients), and (again, in some cases) they may provide an increasing amount of free care. But what does this all mean for their level of professional satisfaction, which plays into their own expectations about the delivery of health care? The literature evaluating physician satisfaction reports large regional variations but an overall trend of decreasing job satisfaction (Zuger, 2004). Such mounting dissatisfaction may lead to poor clinical patient management, the practice of defensive medicine, rapid turnover at hospitals, and, therefore, compromised patient coordination (DiMatteo et al., 1993; Fitzgibbons, Bordley, Berkowitz, Miller, & Henderson, 2006; Haas et al., 2000; Mello et al., 2004; Pathman et al., 2002; Zuger, 2004).

3.3 WELLNESS AS A MOVING TARGET: READING THE EXPECTATIONS OF THE MANY STAKEHOLDERS

Medical information may come from a variety of sources, including legitimate news media reports that typically evaluate published results of scientific inquiry. Filling the health information space are flyers, leaflets, Web sites and portals designed by drug and device companies, and other stakeholders in the health care industry. The purpose, claim the pharmaceutical companies, is to educate patients. Without a doubt, such information is useful to patients and consumers, but these sources are often perceived as having a bias and are designed to promote a particular treatment among both providers and patients who may, in turn, direct business toward the sale of a drug or device treatment. These materials, both printed and online, may even take on the guise of news, medical publications, or government-like health guidelines, so it is not surprising that readers of this information are unclear as to a hidden agenda to sell a product. There is also a seemingly endless supply of opinionated information sources, such as editorial columns appearing in newspapers, magazines, and scientific journals, as well as a growing number of social media Web sites and blogs that peddle information in return for the advertising dollars or the promotion of a particular medical society.

It goes without saying that not all readers of health-related information are able to distinguish a carefully sourced news article from an opinion piece supposedly written by a doctor but actually paid for and generated by a particular medical society or drug company. All this aside, it is important to note that when it comes to health, the news media is another important stakeholder vying for attention. For the most part, developers of drugs or devices are happy to receive media attention when it helps promote their research both within and outside of their university or institution, so their expectation is for positive publicity. Many of the same stakeholders, however, may attack or criticize the news media when negative findings are published and then brought to the public's attention in eye-catching headlines.

In Section 3.2 we wrote about the patients' changing notions of wellness. Expectations about wellness and health also have an influence on the way the payers sponsor health care. If, for example, an employee has type 2 diabetes, he or she may be predisposed to a lot of small, preventable health problems. However, the patient's employer may want to take a larger stake in keeping him or her healthy, so as to limit both absenteeism and presenteeism. In the past, perhaps, diabetes was seen as yet another chronic health problem. These days, some employers are taking extra steps to make sure their diabetic employees are aware of good diabetic care, so as to limit the expenses associated with treating acute problems associated with a poorly managed chronic illness. Other employers, however, may want to divest themselves of the expenses associated with paying for medical care, as these costs are seen as burdensome. There are very different and notable trends among stakeholders that take a role in making private health payments through benefits packages. This is a key area that we explore in Chapter 7.

Providers are also riding a wave of changing notions of wellness, much of the shift in expectations having occurred due to thinking related to preventative medicine. There has been growing pressure to prevent chronic conditions before they occur. This can lead to better outcomes, and indeed plenty of evidence backs up the notion of early treatment leading to better outcomes. The result is that doctors may prescribe medicines earlier. High cholesterol, for example, is treated more aggressively today (Grundy et al., 2004), as is osteoporosis (Kroth, Murray, & McDonald, 2004), and in some cases type 2 diabetes is treated quite successfully with gastric bypass surgery (Buchwald et al., 2009), which was once considered as an extreme measure only to curb morbid obesity.

Certainly, early detection is the key to prevention and to meeting our expectations for better outcomes. Finding earlier warning signs for disease, such as metabolic syndrome, can slow or prevent the progress of diabetes and other common comorbidities like obesity, high blood pressure, and even heart disease (Pi-Sunyer, 2007). But not all tests designed to detect disease at an early stage have had a positive impact on bringing down the morbidity or mortality rate of the disease burden. Recently, controversy surrounded the administration of a widely used screening exam for prostate cancer known as the PSA test. This test looks for prostate-specific antigen, thought to be a key marker for prostate cancer and/or the inflammation believed to be a hallmark of cancer. Two landmark studies showed that screening men for prostate cancer with this test did not necessarily lead to better outcomes such as fewer deaths (Andriole et al., 2009; Schroder et al., 2009). To make matters worse, those interpreting the evidence presented in these two studies believe that many men might have undergone treatment and surgeries that were unnecessary and potentially injurious, with common side effects such as impotency and incontinence (Kolata, 2009).

This begs the question of whether costs spent on treatment and diagnostics can be measured and then justified. The FDA is tasked with the safety of drugs, procedures, and devices, but as of yet it cannot make accurate assessments about whether a given procedure is worth the cost. Many Americans may view the idea of asking government to decide whether a particular health treatment is worthwhile for a particular patient as particularly distasteful, or even unethical. For many other stakeholder groups, limiting the use of a drug or device due to high cost is something only the market should do, not government.

Yet in some countries where taxpayers foot the health care bills almost entirely through a government-run single-payer system, asking if a treatment is worth the cost is part and parcel of business. In the United Kingdom, which has a single-payer system, a British government agency known as the National Institute for Health and Clinical Excellence (NICE) was conceived simply to figure out which treatments are worthy of funding (Harris, 2008). NICE came to fruition in the era of Viagra, when British policy makers feared that the costs of this new blockbuster erectile-dysfunction drug could bankrupt the UK health care system. The agency's goal was simple: it measured the cost-to-quality ratio of every treatment and device and then decided what was worthy or unworthy of the publicly funded expense. But years into its existence, NICE drew great controversy when a kidney cancer patient was denied a drug that promised to extend his life by six months (Harris, 2008). The popular press in the United Kingdom interpreted the decision in these stark terms: the six extra months of life for this individual were not worth the government expense for the medicine.

Despite the public outrage that followed this and other individual cases in the United Kingdom, some U.S. policy makers have looked into adopting similar practices that would curb the costs of medicines and treatment thought of as excessive (Harris, 2008). Perhaps particularly unpalatable to U.S. doctors, hospitals, insurers, policy makers, and patients themselves is the idea of a less empowered patient. The now iconic "Harry and Louise" advertising campaign, funded by the insurance industry in 1993, criticized the Clinton health reforms by playing into such fears (Toner, 1994). In one ad, a white, middle-class American couple (played by hired actors) sits at a kitchen table (Toner). The screen flashes to "sometime in the future," and we see Harry and Louise mulling over changes to their health insurance plan, theoretically brought on by the Clinton administration health reform. "This was covered in our old health plan," says Louise; "Yeah, that was a good one, wasn't it," says Harry. A narrator's voice comes next, saying: "Things are changing, and not for the better; the government is forcing us to pick from a few health care plans designed by government bureaucrats" (Singer, 2009).

The original ad campaign was effective, and many implicate it in the derailment of the Clinton health reforms (Lieberman, 2008; Toner, 1994). The major flaw in the Clinton health reform package was that it excluded so many major stakeholders from the reform process. Because expectations from stakeholding parties were not taken into account, it was not surprising that the only consensus on reform among many constituents was that it should not happen. Quite surprisingly, the Harry and Louise characters made a comeback recently, but this time they starred in an ad campaign supporting health reform (Lieberman, 2008; Singer, 2009). The campaign was funded by a rather unexpected alliance of stakeholders, which includes (but is not limited to) the American Cancer Society's Action Network, the American Hospital Association, the Catholic Health Association, Families USA, and the National Federation of Independent Business (Lieberman, 2008; Singer, 2009). The president of the current industry association for insurers—the American Health Insurance Plans (AHIP)—also made an appearance at a press conference announcing the ad campaign, but this time the insurers are not the major sponsor. (To see the clips of the old and new Harry and Louise campaigns, visit the online version of Natasha Singer's *New York Times* article "Harry and Louise Return, With a New Message," available at http://www.nytimes.com/2009/07/17/business/media/17adco.html, and follow the embedded YouTube video links).

What became stunningly clear was that many stakeholders agree that some sort of fix to the skyrocketing costs and diminishing access to health care is required. Hence, we have the passing of the watered-down Health Care and Education Reconciliation Act of 2010. We cannot blame the government for the problems that this reform bill attempts to tackle, as we do not have a single-payer system; nor can we lay the blame on the insurers who face the business challenge of trying to maintain coverage and quality at affordable prices, or the employers who in tough economic times are struggling to keep workers with benefits on their books. The blame cannot fall on the providers—many hospitals, for example, operate with thin margins or annual shortfalls. We ask whether the patients are to blame. To this question, many say of course not; patients do not choose to be elderly or sick. However, patients are not entirely free from responsibility: we see a clear trend of patients who simply give up on maintaining their health.

The point we are driving at here is that there are no single stakeholders who can, or should, shoulder the blame for problems felt by one or another stakeholder in the U.S. health care system. Every stakeholder owns a part of the health care crisis, and by this same reasoning every stakeholder owns a part of the health care restructuring effort. Again, we see our apt analogy of the Gordian knot, with the tangle in the center only growing deeper as the stakeholders pull on the twine from all angles.

3.4 STAKEHOLDER ALIGNMENT AND THE CREATION OF VALUE

What are the chances that our health care will improve? There are big changes afoot. However, those changes are unlikely to fully succeed unless stakeholder alignment is achieved. Merely solving a cost issue does not necessarily mean we are going to have improved quality, just as simply providing better access to coverage does not mean we are going to decrease poor outcomes. Even if all the stakeholders agree that we need to enable wider access to coverage; eliminate medical errors; stitch together a better continuum of care; and ensure that the cost of providing care remains affordable for the employers, government, and others, such an agreement would not necessarily translate into stakeholder alignment. For so many stakeholders in health care, it is practically inconceivable that alignment might be achievable. So we ask the question: why is alignment so difficult? To answer this we may glimpse at history for answers.

We can examine why past reforms might have failed—and it is undeniable that the history of undertaking health care reform in the United States is littered with failure. Teddy Roosevelt proposed a comprehensive national health system, and that failed. Franklin D. Roosevelt proposed a medical care overhaul as part of the New Deal; those reforms got axed at the very last minute in the 1930s. FDR decided to sacrifice the health coverage portion of his proposed reforms to make his New Deal agenda more attractive to its opponents (Birn, Brown, Fee, & Lear, 2003; Hoffman, 2003). A national medical insurance program was proposed during the Truman era. The American Medical Association first lent tentative support for President Truman's idea, only to reverse their position and successfully oppose the legislation, condemning it in Cold War rhetoric as "socialized medicine." Both Eisenhower and Johnson proposed comprehensive systems, and Johnson only succeeded with Medicare as a part of the Social Security Act following Kennedy's assassination (Birn et al., 2003; Hoffman, 2003). Nixon, of all people, proposed a type of nationalized health insurance—a single-payer system—which, perhaps because of its timing, went nowhere (Birn et al., 2003). Then there were the reform measures proposed by the Clinton administration, which failed amid plans that basically excluded a great number of stakeholders from weighing in on possible health care delivery improvement. In recent times we have the passing of President Obama's Health Care and Education Reconciliation Act of 2010, and we have yet to witness the role it will take in enabling positive change.

Here in the United States, we have a history of several things. We have a history of big ideas and a strongly felt need for reform, and even a history of some concrete solutions. Solutions have been undercut by stakeholders often enough to result in a lack of confidence and trust in the other stakeholding parties. So long as there is a conflict or the possibility of a zero-sum game, and with that the perception that your extra dollar comes directly out of my pocket, nothing will get fixed. This book is about rethinking, and it is about reevaluating. We may learn lessons from history, but that does not guarantee that we will find stakeholder alignment to improve health care delivery going forward. This is especially true if the stakeholders do not expect to align their expectations. Until there emerges a trust, and therefore an expectation that alignment is the key to bringing about change, we will not have a long-term plan, or even a simple way forward. We have arrived at our central argument again: stakeholder cooperation is the key to value creation, regardless of the form and shape health care reform takes.

REFERENCES

Ahluwalia, I. B., & Bolen, J. (2008). Lack of health insurance coverage among working-age adults, evidence from the Behavioral Risk Factor Surveillance System, 1993–2006. *Journal of Community Health, 33*(5), 293–296.

Andriole, G. L., R. L. Grubb, 3rd, et al. (2009). Mortality results from a randomized prostate-cancer screening trial. *New England Journal of Medicine.*

Barlow, P. (1999). Health care is not a human right. *British Medical Journal, 319* (7205), 321.

Berwick, D., Davidoff, F., Hiatt, H., & Smith, R. (2001). Refining and implementing the Tavistock principles for everybody in health care. *British Medical Journal, 323*(7313), 616–620.

Berwick, D., Hiatt, H., Janeway, P., & Smith, R. (1997). An ethical code for everybody in health care. *British Medical Journal, 315*(7123), 1633–1634.

Birn, A. E., Brown, T. M., Fee, E., & Lear, W. J. (2003). Struggles for national health reform in the United States. *American Journal of Public Health, 93*(1), 86–91.

Buchwald, H., Estok, R., Fahrbach, K., Banel, D., Jensen, M. D., Pories, W. J., et al. (2009). Weight and type-2 diabetes after bariatric surgery: Systematic review and meta-analysis. *American Journal of Medicine, 122*(3), 248–256 e245.

Chernew, M., Cutler, D. M., & Keenan, P. S. (2005). Increasing health insurance costs and the decline in insurance coverage. *Health Services Research, 40*(4), 1021–1039.

Cohen, R. A., Martinez, M. E., & Ward, B. W. (2010). *Health insurance coverage: Early release of estimates from the National Health Interview Survey, 2009* [Electronic version]. Retrieved July 15, 2010, from http://www.cdc.gov/nchs/nhis.htm

Collins, S. R., & Nicholson, J. L. (2010). *Rite of Passage: Young adults and the Affordable Care Act of 2010* [Issue brief]. Retrieved January 5, 2011, from http://www.commonwealthfund.org/~/media/Files/Publications/Issue%20Brief/2010/May/1404_Collins_rite_of_passage_2010_v3.pdf

Commonwealth Fund. (2008). National scorecard on health system performance, 2008 [Electronic version]. Retrieved July 13, 2010, from http://www.commonwealthfund.org/usr_doc/site_docs/slideshows/NatlScorecard/NatlScorecard.html

The Commonwealth Fund Commission on a High Performance Health System. (2008). Why not the best? Results from the national scorecard on U.S. health system performance, 2008 [Electronic version]. Retrieved July 13, 2010, from #http://www.commonwealthfund.org/Content/Publications/Fund-Reports/2008/Jul/Why-Not-the-Best-Results-from-the-National-Scorecard-on-U-S–Health-System-Performance–2008.aspx

The Commonwealth Fund. (2009). The Commonwealth Fund Survey of Young Adults: 2009. Retrieved from #http://www.commonwealthfund.org/Content/Surveys/2009/Dec/The-Commonwealth-Fund-Survey-of-Young-Adults.aspx

Cummins, R. O., Smith, R. W., & Inui, T. S. (1980). Communication failure in primary care. Failure of consultants to provide follow-up information. *Journal of the American Medical Association, 243*(16), 1650–1652.

Davis, K., Schoen, C., Doty, M., & Tenney, K. (2002). Medicare vs. private insurance: Rhetoric and reality. *Health Affairs (Millwood)*, Web Exclusives, w311–w324.

DeNavas-Walt, C., Proctor, B. D., & Smith, J. C. (2008). *Income, Poverty, and Health Insurance Coverage in the United States: 2008*. Washington, DC: U.S. Census Bureau.

DiMatteo, M. R., Sherbourne, C. D., Hays, R. D., Ordway, L., Kravitz, R. L., McGlynn, E. A., et al. (1993). Physicians' characteristics influence patients' adherence to medical treatment: Results from the Medical Outcomes Study. *Journal of Health Psychology, 12*(2), 93–102.

Dranove, D., & Millenson, M. L. (2006). Medical bankruptcy: Myth versus fact. *Health Affairs (Millwood), 25*(2), w74–w83.

Fitzgibbons, J. P., Bordley, D. R., Berkowitz, L. R., Miller, B. W., & Henderson, M. C. (2006). Redesigning residency education in internal medicine: A position paper from the Association of Program Directors in Internal Medicine. *Annals of Internal Medicine, 144*(12), 920–926.

Glied, S., & Mahato, B. (2008). Analysis of the March 2008 Current Population Survey. Retrieved January 5, 2011, from http://www.commonwealthfund.org/~/media/Files/Publications/Testimony/2009/Apr/Testimony%20Young%20and%20Vulnerable/PPT%20and%20PDF/PDF%20City%20Council%20Hearing%204%2023%2009%20Figures%20FINAL.pdf

Grundy, S. M., Cleeman, J. I., Merz, C. N., Brewer, H. B., Jr., Clark, L. T., Hunninghake, D. B., et al. (2004). Implications of recent clinical trials for the National Cholesterol Education Program Adult Treatment Panel III Guidelines. *Journal of the American College of Cardiology, 44*(3), 720–732.

Haas, J. S., Cook, E. F., Puopolo, A. L., Burstin, H. R., Cleary, P. D., & Brennan, T. A. (2000). Is the professional satisfaction of general internists associated with patient satisfaction? *Journal of General Internal Medicine, 15*(2), 122–128.

Hall, A. G., J. S. Harman, et al. (2008). Lapses in medicaid coverage: impact on cost and utilization among individuals with diabetes enrolled in medicaid. *Med Care 46*(12), 1219–1225.

Hall, A. G., C. H. Lemak, et al. (2008). Expanding the definition of access: it isn't just about health insurance. *Journal of Health Care for the Poor and Underserved 19*(2), 625–638.

Hardin, G. (1968). The tragedy of the commons. *Science, 162*(5364), 1243–1248.

Harris, G. (2008). British balance benefit vs. cost of latest drugs. *New York Times*. New York.

Higgins, M. J., Rae, J. M., Flockhart, D. A., Hayes, D. F., & Stearns, V. (2009). Pharmacogenetics of tamoxifen: Who should undergo CYP2D6 genetic testing? *Journal of the National Comprehensive Cancer Network, 7*(2), 203–213.

Higgins, M. J., & Stearns, V. (2009). Understanding resistance to tamoxifen in hormone receptor-positive breast cancer. *Clinical Chemistry, 55*(8), 1453–1455.

Himmelstein, D. U., Warren, E., Thorne, D., & Woolhandler, S. (2005). Illness and injury as contributors to bankruptcy. *Health Affairs (Millwood)*, Web Exclusives, w5-63–w5-73.

Himmelstein, D. U., Woolhandler, S., & Wolfe, S. M. (1992). The vanishing health care safety net: New data on uninsured Americans. *International Journal of Health Services, 22*(3), 381–396.

Hoffman, B. (2003). Health care reform and social movements in the United States. *American Journal of Public Health, 93*(1), 75–85.

Jencks, S. F., Williams, M. V., & Coleman, E. A. (2009). Rehospitalizations among patients in the Medicare fee-for-service program. *New England Journal of Medicine, 360*(14), 1418–1428.

Jenkins, C. L. (2008, March 18). Unwelcome surprise: Fairfax doctors' shift to boutique care leaves patients weighing options. *Washington Post*. Retrieved December 1, 2010, from http://www.washingtonpost.com/wp-dyn/content/article/2008/03/14/AR2008031403519_2.html

Keith, A. (2000). The economics of Viagra. *Health Affairs (Millwood), 19*(2), 147–157.

Kennedy, J., Tuleu, I., & Mackay, K. (2008). Unfilled prescriptions of Medicare beneficiaries: Prevalence, reasons, and types of medicines prescribed. *Journal of Managed Care Pharmacy, 14*(6), 553–560.

Klein, K., Glied, S., & Ferry, D. (2005). Entrances and exits: Health insurance churning, 1998–2000 [Electronic version]. *Issue Brief (Commonwealth Fund)*, 1–12. Abstract retrieved September 1, 2009, from http://www.ncbi.nlm.nih.gov/entrez/query.fcgi?cmd=Retrieve&db=PubMed&dopt=Citation&list_uids=16180284

Kolata, G. (2009, March 19). Prostate test found to save few lives. *New York Times*, p. A1.

Kripalani, S., LeFevre, F., Phillips, C. O., Williams, M. V., Basaviah, P., & Baker, D. W. (2007). Deficits in communication and information transfer between hospital-based and primary care physicians: Implications for patient safety and continuity of care. *Journal of the American Medical Association, 297*(8), 831–841.

Lieberman, T. (2008). Harry and Louise are back again: But the media miss the important subtext. *Columbia Journalism Review*.

Leininger, L. J. (2009). Partial-year insurance coverage and the health care utilization of children. *Med Care Res Rev 66*(1), 49–67.

Lenzer, J. (2008). Underinsurance threatens physical and financial wellbeing of US families. *Bmj 336*(7658): 1399.

Kroth, P. J., Murray, M. D., & McDonald, C. J. (2004). Undertreatment of osteoporosis in women, based on detection of vertebral compression fractures on chest radiography. *American Journal of Geriatric Pharmacotherapy, 2*(2), 112–118.

Mello, M. M., Studdert, D. M., DesRoches, C. M., Peugh, J., Zapert, K., Brennan, T. A., et al. (2004). Caring for patients in a malpractice crisis: Physician satisfaction and quality of care. *Health Affairs (Millwood), 23*(4), 42–53.

Moore, C., Wisnivesky, J., Williams, S., & McGinn, T. (2003). Medical errors related to discontinuity of care from an inpatient to an outpatient setting. *Journal of General Internal Medicine, 18*(8), 646–651.

O'Donnell, H. C., Kaushal, R., Barron, Y., Callahan, M. A., Adelman, R. D., & Siegler, E. L. (2009). Physicians' attitudes towards copy and pasting in electronic note writing. *Journal of General Internal Medicine, 24*(1), 63–68.

Oswald, D. P., J. N. Bodurtha, et al. (2007). Underinsurance and key health outcomes for children with special health care needs. *Pediatrics, 119*(2), e341–347.

Pathman, D. E., Konrad, T. R., Williams, E. S., Scheckler, W. E., Linzer, M., & Douglas, J. (2002). Physician job satisfaction, dissatisfaction, and turnover. *Journal of Family Practice, 51*(7), 593.

Pi-Sunyer, X. (2007). The metabolic syndrome: How to approach differing definitions. *Medical Clinics of North America, 91*(6), 1025–1040, vii.

Pollack, A. (2008, December 30). Patient's DNA may be signal to tailor medication. *New York Times*, p. 1.

Pollack, A. (2010, June 12). FDA faults companies on unapproved genetic tests. *New York Times*, p. B2.

Roy, C. L., Poon, E. G., Karson, A. S., Ladak-Merchant, Z., Johnson, R. E., Maviglia, S. M., et al. (2005). Patient safety concerns arising from test results that return after hospital discharge. *Annals of Internal Medicine, 143*(2), 121–128.

Sack, K., & Zezima, K. (2009, January 21). Growing need for Medicaid strains states. *New York Times*, p. A25.

Saunders, M. R., & Alexander, G. C. (2009). Turning and churning: Loss of health insurance among adults in Medicaid. *Journal of General Internal Medicine, 24*(1), 133–134.

Schoen, C., & Osborn, R. (2004). *The Commonwealth Fund 2004 international health policy survey of primary care in five countries* [Chartpack]. Retrieved December 2, 2010, from The Commonwealth Fund website: http://bit.ly/hIEY10

Seifert, R. W., & Rukavina, M. (2006). Bankruptcy is the tip of a medical-debt iceberg. *Health Affairs (Millwood), 25*(2), w89–w92.

Singer, N. (2009, July 17). Harry and Louise return, with a new message. *New York Times*, p. B3.

Smith, R., Hiatt, H., & Berwick, D. (1999). Shared ethical principles for everybody in health care: A working draft from the Tavistock group. *British Medical Journal, 318*(7178), 248–251.

Toner, R. (1994, September 30). Harry and Louise and a guy named Ben. *New York Times*. Retrieved December 1, 2010, from http://www.nytimes.com/1994/09/30/us/harry-and-louise-and-a-guy-named-ben.html

U.S. Census Bureau. (2010). *Income, poverty, and health insurance coverage in the United States: 2009* [Report]. (Publication No. P60–238). Retrieved December 2, 2010, from http://www.census.gov/hhes/www/hlthins/data/incpovhlth/2009/highlights.html

Wolters Kluwer Health (2009). 2008 sees significant rise in prescription abandonment and uptake of generics. Bridgewater, NJ.

Zuger, A. (2004). Dissatisfaction with medical practice. *New England Journal of Medicine, 350*(1), 69–75.

Zuger, A. (2005, October 30). For a retainer, lavish care by "boutique doctors." *New York Times*. Retrieved December 1, 2010, from http://www.nytimes.com/2005/10/30/health/30patient.html

4 Stakeholders in Health Care: A Field Guide to Identification and Evaluation

4.1 DEFINING STAKEHOLDERS: WHO ARE THEY? WHO ARE YOU? WHO ARE WE?

One illuminating exercise I use with health care professionals is to ask them to identify the major stakeholders by first taking a look at how they define themselves. We then go on to look at where the different groups stand on a variety of issues; we go about this task as if we were anthropologists building a field guide to a yet-unexplored landscape. Throughout history, humans have handed down guides (some oral, some pictorial, and some written) to serve as collections of information that may help subsequent explorers navigate the unfamiliar. But, make no mistake, field guides are often interpretative, a hallmark trait being that the narrator imprints his or her own impressions on a generation of explorers that follow. It is no surprise, then, that the contemporary field guide may be more of an amalgamation of different perspectives, rather than the perspective of an individual narrator.

We live in the era of Wikipedia, where many individuals contribute bits of information which are then debated, edited, rewritten, and consolidated into a more global view. Wikipedia is an example of one resource that is user-generated and updated at regular intervals, providing a snapshot of ideas that are forever evolving. As we are all well aware, any particular entry in Wikipedia can provide information that is concise yet, sometimes, irrelevant. As in other encyclopedias, it can also include biases and inaccuracies. Unlike other encyclopedias, though, Wikipedia struggles from time to time with "vandal" users who maliciously feed inaccuracies into an entry (Boudreau & Lakhani, 2009). We encourage our readers to continually update and challenge their previous knowledge of health care stakeholders when making evaluations. But we also want our readers to ask themselves how they might rule out information that is irrelevant, or simply wrong. How can we constantly update our point of view without introducing biases? In this chapter we first work through an example of finding the information pertinent to defining stakeholder groups. Second, we use our taxonomic approach to research the salience of a stakeholder group. Last, we look at how various health care stakeholders may be stymied by their own managerial approach, which typically disregards the other stakeholders in their immediate ecology.

Defining stakeholders, evaluating stakeholder salience, and understanding all the stakeholders' perspectives are important steps toward reaching stakeholder alignment. This is a valuable approach not only because this methodology helps various stakeholders get a better grasp of one another's interests and expectations, but also because we can begin to decode how information, knowledge, and even talent get warehoused within and among health care stakeholders. The process of warehousing often results in what can be called "silos." The concept of silos has been described in the broader business literature, and in recent years the notion has been used to help characterize some of the major shortcomings in the sharing of information in health care. These silos exist in small and large entities within hospitals, for example. But silos are found between and within large stakeholder groups, too (e.g., the many types of payers and the various types of providers). However, before going on to discuss silos, we will first focus on defining stakeholders.

4.2 UNDERSTANDING THE LIMITATIONS IN DEFINING STAKEHOLDER GROUPS

In the spirit of our anthropological approach, I put groups to task, asking them to come up with and then edit a contemporary field guide for health care. Participants start with basic questions about stakeholder groups, which are lumped into larger, all-encompassing categories. What follows is a simple guide I give to my students: I ask them to start with a simple "mega" category, like "patients" or "payers," and expand from there. When we look at the group that is sometimes called providers, we warn participants to take extra care: hospitals and physician groups can be as different as night and day. It is somewhat unfortunate that they are often lumped together. Payers, too, include employers, government, and the patient; these are very different types of payers, with different agendas, expectations, and power.

I give participants a chart to follow. This is an exercise that needs both time and careful consideration. We urge participants to undertake a literature search and make time to discuss the findings, as this is typically done as a group assignment (we believe the results may be more insightful when individuals work together).

If you refer to Figure 4.1, you can see that we first ask participants to begin with Step 1 and answer the question: "What is out there?" We then go on to ask them to name the major groups and subgroups and to select one group. It is at this point that the real thought for this exercise begins. Quickly, participants find that they would like to create a series of subgroups and categories that, when taken together,

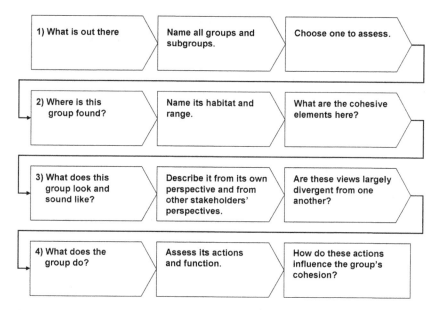

FIGURE 4.1 The taxonomic approach.

may seem oddly appropriated into the same bucket. Participants often start out with dictionary definitions but quickly disagree on how well or how badly these definitions characterize a group. Let us look for a moment at the group commonly referred to as "patients." The Merriam-Webster online dictionary defines a patient as "an individual awaiting or under medical care and treatment" or "the recipient of any of various personal services," or, finally, "one that is acted upon" (Merriam-Webster Online, 2009) The online version of the *Oxford English Dictionary* defines a patient as "a person receiving or registered to receive medical treatment" (Oxford Dictionaries Online, 2009).

The latter definition captures the notion of an intention to treat but makes it clear that the individual does not necessarily have to receive any treatment in order to be categorized as a patient. One vice president of a nursing institution suggested that these definitions seem to imply that once an individual becomes a patient there is a certain loss of power, or passiveness. Many students, in reading though contemporary literature, point out that the patient is very often referred to as a consumer or a customer. These are words that suggest there is choice and power and, of course, an exchange of money involved. The word "patient" alone does not necessarily capture this aspect, so sometimes we see in the literature the compound phrase "patient-consumer."

It is at this point that we typically enter into a polemical discussion about the merits and pitfalls of consumer-driven health care. We will spare our readers such a discussion, as debating this point is not the intent of the exercise or the goal of this book. Suffice to say that the providers and payers, both public and private, and the patients themselves sometimes use the word "consumer" to connote "patient." In the literature this usage appeared with increasing frequency in the mid-1970s.

Patients have been called "consumers" whether they have a lot or little choice, information, access, and/or resources to a share in services provided in the realm of health care. Putting the literature aside for now, patients and other stakeholders occasionally choose to use other words instead of patient. These sentiments have been summarized well in the Wikipedia definition of the word "patient," particularly under the subheading "alternative terminology" (Wikipedia, 2009).

Other terms that are sometimes used include health consumer, health care consumer or client. These may be used by governmental agencies, insurance companies, patient groups, or health care facilities. Individuals who use or have used psychiatric services may alternatively refer to themselves as consumers, users, or survivors. In nursing homes and assisted living facilities, the term resident is generally used in lieu of patient, but it is not uncommon for staff members at such a facility to use the term patient in reference to residents.

Similarly, those receiving home health care are called "clients" (Wikipedia, 2009).

Since Wikipedia is constantly being updated and edited by numerous people, we encourage our readers to look up the latest definition. We believe it offers a window to some of our contemporary sentiments about being a patient. Perhaps we would add to it that many different types of patients (not just psychiatric patients) refer to themselves as "survivors." For example, we often hear the phrase "cancer survivor" used to describe patients whose cancer has gone into remission. The word "survivor" suggests a regaining of power following a struggle. As one medical director suggested, it has a far less passive tone than the word "patient." Also, we want to add that at any given time an individual may not want to use the word "patient" to describe himself or herself. Some may choose to define themselves as health consumers with a degree of choice and power rather than patients with a health problem.

Many times when we have had heated discussions about what, if anything, differentiates a patient from a consumer, a number of health care professionals seem to agree on one single point: how an individual acts and defines himself or herself can also influence the way other stakeholders around that person act. This may be a universal truth that does not apply only to individuals. During this exercise we encourage our participants to go to the Web sites of their major stakeholders and read the mission statements of the institutions and entities within these groups. Surprisingly, mission statements can be curiously revealing, not only for what they include, but also for what they do not include. Take the Centers for Medicare and Medicaid (CMS), the government entity that manages government-sponsored health insurance programs. Emerging and existing health care leaders alike are surprised to learn that CMS's mission statement does not include a pledge to improve upon health outcomes, but instead offers to "ensure effective, up-to-date healthcare coverage and to promote quality care for beneficiaries" (Centers for Medicare and Medicaid Services [CMS], 2009).

Similarly, Aetna, the private insurer, avoided the issue of improving upon health outcomes for its participants. We accessed their mission statement on the company

Web page under a section subtitled, "Why We Exist: The Aetna Mission." In this mission statement there was much written about delivering "safe, cost-effective, high-quality health care" to people while "protecting their finances against health-related risks" (Aetna, 2009). The company talks about cooperating with providers like doctors and hospitals as well as patients and public officials to "build a stronger, more effective health care system" (Aetna, 2009). As some of our participants noted, there was nothing said about improving health outcomes or promoting preventative medicine. Hospitals are also an interesting stakeholder group, as many of them were founded as charitable organizations. Many hospitals have long since abandoned their nonprofit roots, yet they have continued to fundraise and hang on to charity-oriented sentiment in their mission statements. We sifted through about a dozen mission statements to find that while quality care and patient satisfaction were often mentioned, only a handful spoke of actually improving upon the health of their patrons.

Massachusetts General Hospital is one such hospital, offering a succinct mission statement that promises to "improve the health and well-being of the diverse communities we serve." This mission is the product of recent revisions made to better reflect a continued promise to care for Boston's "sick poor," as was originally envisioned over 200 years ago by the hospital's founders (Quinlan, 2008). Other hospitals pledge first "to discover," "to teach," and "to learn," and to make "world-class contributions"; yet human health was also to be at "the center of academic culture" (NYU Langone Medical Center, 2009). We see a great number of mission statements that pledge to put the patient at "the center," and still more offer "compassion" and "respect" to patients. One hospital system, Banner Health, which serves areas in both Arizona and Alaska, states, "We show value results by exceeding the expectations of the people we serve, as well as the expectations we set for ourselves" (Banner Health, 2009). This begs at least two questions: who is setting these service and health expectations, and do these expectations start off with high or low hopes?

The point being made here is that stakeholders are defined, in great part, by their history and the perception they have of themselves. The experience of reading through mission statements serves to remind us that all stakeholders in health care come from a unique perspective. Understanding or being aware of this perspective, at least in part, is also a major step in identifying the stakeholder groups and subgroups. However, this is just one part of the exercise. It is a sort of a warm-up exercise. At this point I am going to share an example of how I, with student-participant input, went about defining a single stakeholder group through a more extensive examination of academic literature, media reports, editorials and speeches from key opinion leaders, and statements from other stakeholders.

Importantly, I tell my students to go about this exercise by first eliminating any biases and preconceived ideas they hold about the stakeholder groups they are researching, and to start this search as if they know nothing or very little about the stakeholder group. Section 4.3 reveals some of the literature our students and executive education participants recently reviewed as they completed the chart that appears in Figure 4.1. It does not detail every piece of literature we retrieved, but it does reflect the rigor with which we use our anthropological method to create a salient picture of one particular stakeholder.

4.3 STAKEHOLDER SALIENCE IN THE HEALTH CARE WORLD

Stakeholder saliency has come to mean a number of different things. Typically, a "stakeholder saliency" exercise is used by one stakeholder to assess the other stakeholders in its immediate vicinity. This may be achieved by earnest evaluations of each group's power, legitimacy, and urgency to influence or achieve a certain agenda (Mitchell, Agle, & Wood, 1997). For now we are not going to evaluate these items directly or individually in regard to actions. Instead we urge our readers to note, in this chapter, when influence is discussed and how this relates to the power and legitimacy of this particular stakeholder. In coming chapters we will endeavor to lead our readers through a stakeholder-mapping process. For now we will continue with this exercise, which introduces stakeholder salience through our taxomonic approach.

We started with the category "hospitals," for which we named the various types of descriptive categories found in the United States: teaching, public municipal, community, faith-based, rural, suburban, specialty hospitals, rehabilitative, ambulatory surgery centers, and military/VA hospitals. This list of types of hospitals is not all-inclusive, and there is some overlap. For example, a rural hospital may also be considered a community hospital. Perhaps because some of our participants had also trained as clinicians, they decided to narrow in on "teaching hospitals," which are sometimes also referred to as "academic hospitals" or "university hospitals." Here we caution them, because while all academic hospitals may be teaching hospitals, not all teaching hospitals are affiliated with a single university or college. Many military or VA teaching hospitals affiliate with more than one medical school (United States Department of Veterans Affairs, 2009). However, a great number of teaching hospitals may be owned by a medical school, while a smaller proportion of medical schools, including Harvard Medical School, do not own a single hospital and instead affiliate with numerous area hospitals (Garvin & Roberto, 2002). According to one teaching-hospital Web site, training, research, and patient care are three typically interrelated pursuits with obvious commonalities (Duke University Health System [DUHS], 2009).

In our classes and executive education programs, I challenge students and participants to explain in detail what these commonalities mean. They point out that a lot of teaching hospitals are found in cities, where they also serve as urban safety-net hospitals. In addition to functioning as centers for research and training, safety-net hospitals also provide care for the uninsured and Medicaid-reliant populations (National Association of Urban Hospitals [NAUH], 2009). They went on to add that many teaching hospitals are not only affiliated with a university but may also be physically attached or close to major medical schools. Their cohesive element is that these institutions train the more than 100,000 medical residents who eventually become physicians and other types of medical staff serving all over the United States. Another element is that they often have facilities to treat rare diseases, as well as specialized trauma centers that offer expertise with severe or complicated problems, such as serious burn injuries (Association of American Medical Colleges [AAMC], 2010). A great majority of teaching hospitals will also conduct research that is typically sponsored by both the public and private sectors.

Teaching hospitals also comprise components of other stakeholder groups in health care. They may be extensions of large government agencies such as the National Institutes of Health (NIH), or they may be a component of the NIH, such as the National Cancer Institute (NCI, 2010). They may even be independent nonprofit institutes and consortiums that receive funding from the private sector as well as grants from other institutions, government, or universities, such as the Center for Integration of Medicine and Innovative Technology (CIMIT, 2009). Research funding can also come directly from pharmaceutical, medical device, or biotechnology firms. This type of funding can take many different forms, one being the funding of basic science, while other funds are allocated for clinical trials designed to investigate the safety and efficacy of a new drug, treatment, or device. Clinical trials may be supported and funded by both private and public money (NCI, 2010). While teaching hospitals are the most common sites for clinical trials, this type of research is not exclusive to teaching hospitals. It is simply that many teaching hospitals are well positioned for the assembly of research expertise and institutional review boards needed for the ethical conduct of such research.

I often point out that the leadership at teaching hospitals may be very high profile—especially for large teaching hospitals attached to medical schools. I ask my students and seminar participants: *"What does this mean for other stakeholders?"* To this question I do not get immediate replies; rather, I get more questions in return. Eventually, some decide that the leadership of a teaching hospital can have a large impact on managing other stakeholders. To try and figure out what this means, a marketing vice president researched the leadership of large teaching hospitals. She saw immediately that they were often quoted in the press, but also that they came under a lot of scrutiny from other stakeholders and the public in general. She pulled from the following examples to demonstrate her point.

A case study written in the words of Paul Levy about his rise to the position of CEO of Beth Israel Deaconess Medical Center demonstrates how academic hospital leadership can change the landscape of a city's health care system. The case study reveals the inner battles of a struggling hospital merger in the Boston area, and how it was rescued with a new vision by new leadership. The account, however, is from the perspective of the leader himself (Garvin & Roberto, 2002). Our stakeholders, including groups that reside within the merged hospitals, may have very different perspectives on what the problems were and what was achieved once Levy took over. The point here is that when they do read the editorials and case studies generated by the leaders of teaching hospitals, they need to understand these leaders offer accounts from their own restricted points of view that these leaders may hold. Such biases aside, words from the leadership can give great insight into the institution itself.

Once the students or participants have examined how the leadership in teaching hospitals characterize their own hospitals, we move on to examine how they interact with and comment on their fellow teaching hospitals. The debate over why Medicaid spending varies among teaching hospitals has sparked many comments from outsiders and those leaders within teaching hospitals. This ongoing debate attracted the poignant comments of the head of the Mayo Clinic, headquartered in Rochester, Minnesota. The Mayo Clinic's network includes a hospital system with teaching facilities and groups of medical practices that are concentrated in Minnesota, Iowa, and Wisconsin, but there are also Mayo Clinic–owned practices in other states such as Florida and Arizona. The president, Dr. Denis A. Cortese, was quoted in the *New York Times* as saying that over the course of a year Medicare wastes billions of dollars because it "pays the most to health care providers and geographic areas that provide the lowest-quality care at the highest costs" (Pear, 2009). In other interviews, Dr. Cortese suggests that many doctors are taught to practice medicine with an intensive approach that requires more spending but does not necessarily improve health outcomes (Wertheimer, 2009). The Mayo Clinic has been held up as an example of health care excellence in the nation, so Dr. Cortese's words do not fall lightly.

Cortese's critics have noted that the Mayo Clinic may be taking credit for better health outcomes that are largely a product of serving a patient population that is not as poor or as diverse as those served by other teaching hospitals (Wertheimer, 2009). Heads of inner city teaching hospitals have long argued that they treat sicker and more challenging Medicare patients. The same *New York Times* article mentioned above also quoted Dr. Steven M. Safyer, president of Montefiore Medical Center in the Bronx. He suggested that his patients often require more intensive medical attention upon arrival, but their poorer outcomes are largely attributable to a lifetime of foregoing medical attention before reaching eligibility for coverage under Medicare (Pear, 2009).

Whether this explanation is true or not is also a matter of great debate. Our health care professionals find that as they review the literature regarding major teaching hospitals, they see very strong trends related to patients' health outcomes. A study looking at health outcomes following all types of surgical procedures shows that surgery patients at major teaching hospitals had lower odds (about a 15% chance) of dying following complications when compared with the odds of dying of the patients receiving surgery at nonteaching hospitals. This benefit was not seen in black patients, however, who had similar odds of dying following surgery complications at both teaching and nonteaching hospitals. One might deduce that the benefits of receiving care at a major teaching hospital are felt only among whites and not among blacks, who receive a disproportionate amount of care at teaching hospitals (Silber et al., 2009).

From this discussion of the literature it is fair to conclude that teaching hospitals occupy an unusual space in our health care ecology. Some students who had not worked near or in a hospital were surprised to learn of the incredible dichotomy that exists within simply defining this large and diverse stakeholder group. The big teaching hospitals are often described as "elite" and as having "cutting-edge" care for rare and enigmatic health problems. Consumer-patients often seek them out for treatment in the hopes of gaining the best care and attention possible. Yet these same hospitals are also tasked with serving the nation's poorest and most neglected patients. So here we begin to understand why the leadership in large teaching hospitals holds substantial political and cultural sway in the wider health care community, yet is the recipient of much critical attention. We also begin to see how some of these leaders are able set the health care agenda for a city or region and leverage their hospital's reputation to influence policy and reimbursement issues.

Some leaders, and by extension the teaching hospitals themselves, have more influence than others, and that influence is often determined by the size and reputation of the institution. Another thing I ask my students to consider is the influence a hospital's leadership can have on reimbursements for patient care and in attracting research funding. Hospitals that are very successful at getting higher reimbursements for patient care and research funding may hold a special regional influence over health care pricing and delivery. A series of investigative reports in the *Boston Globe* outlines how teaching hospitals in the Boston area influence one another and other major stakeholders, such as regional community hospitals, insurers, consumers, and the local government.

One article in particular highlights the differences in reimbursements for the same operation in Boston's teaching hospitals, despite the lack of evidence for higher quality of care among those hospitals. The *Boston Globe*'s team of reporters was able to compare reimbursements among teaching hospitals and between area community hospitals through obtaining private insurance data collected by the Massachusetts Health Care Quality and Cost Council. Some of the comparisons for equivalent care exposed staggering discrepancies in reimbursement. In one case, a teaching hospital was paid 44% more for an operation performed on its premises by a doctor who routinely performs the identical surgery at a lesser-known community hospital (Allen & Bombardieri, 2008).

The article's authors argue that the teaching hospitals that secure the highest reimbursements are the hospitals with the most "clout." The idea of "clout," in essence, translates into reputation and size, which greatly influence the hospital's popularity among consumers. Furthermore, insurers are well aware of the consumer demand for health plans that offer coverage at the teaching hospitals. These patient-consumers, however, are not necessarily informed by actual data demonstrating better care; rather, they are acting on perception (Allen & Bombardieri, 2008). Some competing community hospitals and smaller teaching hospitals complain that they are less well compensated despite having better quality of care than the most highly compensated teaching hospitals in Boston (Allen & Bombardieri, 2008; Allen & Krasner, 2009).

A leader from one of the region's community hospitals argued that the growing reimbursement gap means his hospital is increasingly less able to compete with teaching hospitals on many levels, including doctors' salary, investment in new technology, and inpatient and outpatient capacity (Allen & Bombardieri, 2008). But another leader holding a completely different perspective suggested that teaching hospitals were among the most susceptible to cuts in publicly funded reimbursements. Dr. Darrell Kirch, CEO and president of the Association of American Medical Colleges (AAMC), warned that teaching hospitals that seem able to secure high reimbursements from private-sector payers could easily be targeted for cuts in payment from public funding for Medicare patients. In an appearance during a public health care discussion, he also suggested that cuts to public reimbursements targeted at teaching hospitals could put poorer patients who rely on them in great jeopardy (Kirch, 2009).

There are lots of other supports that flow through Medicare especially toward what are often called the safety-net hospitals. . . . They are also the place where doctors learn their craft. There are a whole series of special Medicare payments that go to those hospitals that have been, at various times, discussed as potential ways to sweep up savings... in my view, again, this would be another cliff we could fall off—to destabilize the safety-net hospitals at a time when we need them as much or as [sic] more than ever.

In the above examples we see plenty of reasons for why teaching hospitals are a rather odd stakeholder group in the wider health care community. They may view one another as natural competitors in the same communities, while also sharing many physicians, technicians, and specialists. No doubt, the teaching hospitals have very different perceptions of themselves and different methods of managing the other stakeholders in their immediate ecology. Still, on the national stage they may act in a far more cohesive manner, issuing statements and press releases that condemn or condone federal moves. For example, in a recent press release the AAMC (2009) thanked the Obama administration for preventing funding cuts to teaching hospitals. Finally, I tell my students and seminar participants that this is fairly typical of many stakeholder groups in health care: they may appear disparate and conflicted from one angle, yet unified and in sync with one another on a national stage.

With this last example we conclude this section on defining stakeholders and stakeholder salience. We feel it unnecessary (even impossible) to define every single health care stakeholder group here, but we encourage readers to use our taxonomic approach to sift through the literature that characterizes, defines, and obscures stakeholder groups in health care. As we mentioned at the beginning of this section, we go into more detail about how stakeholders view one another and themselves in future chapters. But next, we move on to look at silos among and within stakeholders as well as management styles.

4.4 THE SILOS THAT SURROUND US

In business speak, "silos" can be metaphorical towers of information or people holed up within and between stakeholders. These towers develop naturally, in part, through the evolution of performing a particular role. In health care, as in other industries, they may be kept alive intentionally by groups operating within a stakeholder group, as a means of protecting status, job security, and function. That is not to say that they are not often generated unintentionally by inefficiencies or a particular culture, structure, and ecology within the stakeholder community. But when recognized, stakeholders themselves may be well aware that having control over an information silo or talent-based silo can confer great power—and that power is the key to holding influence over other stakeholders. So, for many parties within and among silos, information and operational processes are the key to retaining power.

By this same reasoning, holding on to silos, or keeping them concealed from others, is one strategy for retaining power. Certainly, once silos are revealed they can render the stakeholder less powerful, meaning that there is a disincentive in many instances to make certain information or processes public knowledge. We have already seen this in a number of examples we mentioned earlier. Hospitals may be reluctant to share data on reimbursements, especially when they are well compensated (Allen & Bombardieri, 2008). By the same token, physicians, specialists, and different types of medical communities may also be reluctant to release outcomes data when they feel that their reputation is outpacing their actual performance. There is a body of evidence suggesting that a portion of doctors may resist certain protocols or clinical guidelines (McGlynn, 2003; McGlynn, Kerr, Adams, Keesey, & Asch, 2003), and there have been many editorial reports speculating on why clinical guidelines are often disregarded (de Brantes, Gosfield, McGlynn, Rosenthal, & Levin-Scherz, 2006; Mendelson & Carino, 2005; Steinberg & Luce, 2005).

Insurance firms are reluctant to shed light on why some procedures are covered while others are not in any given coverage plan. My experience is that there is far less transparency in the medical insurance business than, for example, the auto insurance business. Moreover, employers may withhold information about which jobs are worth offering with a pay package that includes health benefits versus jobs that are simply contracted without health benefits. There are many other examples of why different stakeholders keep information from consumers of health care, or from one another. Whatever the individual's or group's motivations behind withholding different types of information, operations, or processes within one area of operation, the result of poor coordination can reflect badly on the stakeholder group as a whole.

A telling study highlighted the existence of silos and a "silo mentality" among groups within a corporation. The study uncovered these silos by analyzing the e-mail communications over a period of time. While this particular corporate entity wanted to encourage the internal sharing of information and talent among employees and groups, the study revealed that natural barriers were the biggest hindrance to communication (Kleinbaum, Stuart, & Tushman, 2008). These silos occurred among working groups and within strategic business units, or between working groups with different organizational functions. But other factors—such as the physical location of workers, gender, and age—were also detected as reasons for silos (Gilbert, 2008; Kleinbaum et al., 2008). In an interview, Toby E. Stuart explained the findings on gender and barriers to information sharing with this fictional scenario:

One can think of it like this. If we were to randomly remove an employee from this company's communication network, the odds that this action would cause a communication breakdown between two units of the company are higher if the employee happened to be female rather than male. Women are more likely than men to link otherwise non-communicating groups of people. (Gilbert, 2008)

In hospitals, for example, silos may be even more pronounced because each group may come from an entirely unique educational and experiential background.

The clinicians themselves represent their own stakeholder group, as do the patients, nurses, administrators, hospital business managers, claim processors, and so on. This is because these groups likely have very different training, academic backgrounds, and work experiences. But they also may share little in common with one another as individuals, and so may never see a reason to communicate with one another if their daily routines and tasks do not force them to.

If silos can yield influence and power through controlling information, they will likely look for ways in which to manage information, talent, and input from other stakeholders. This managing of information can occur at the employee level, where workers decide to not share information outside of their own group. At higher levels this can occur as a strategy to maintain a particular outlook, function, or even image. However, managing information and talent poorly can also result in catastrophic miscalculations and allocation of resources.

A good example of how one stakeholder group is particularly divided on how to handle information was brought to light recently by one of our colleagues, Dr. Tom Delbanco, the Richard and Florence Koplow–James Tullis Professor of General Medicine and Primary Care at Harvard Medical School. He has been trying to persuade physicians to share their own notes with their patients on a regular basis (Knox, 2009; Kowalczyk, 2009). While patients have every legal right to view their medical records, and with them the physicians' notes, they are rarely offered the opportunity to glimpse these insights. Professor Delbanco is suggesting that doctors should be better prepared to share and explain these notes. He also says that he has encountered many barriers to viewing patients' records and notes, such as extra charges (Kowalczyk, 2009). He suggests that those fellow doctors who do not welcome this type of transparency fear such a move would put doctors in danger of more lawsuits from litigious patients. Clinicians fear that they might have to spend too much time explaining notes to patients (Knox, 2009; Kowalczyk, 2009). Some physicians even worry about possibly scaring patients by revealing speculative thoughts about an unconfirmed diagnosis, according to Professor Delbanco (Knox, 2009; Kowalczyk, 2009). However, he also believes that sharing notes with patients will lead to improved patient–physician dialogue and, ultimately, greater understanding (Knox, 2009). Others speculate that this could lead to behavioral changes that foster improved health outcomes, and that in some cases patients might even catch mistakes that would otherwise go unnoticed (Kowalczyk, 2009). Skeptics want evidence that communication would be improved in such a move. Professor Delbanco and his colleagues have launched a formal study whereby patients will get online access to their medical records and doctors notes, but they will also fill out surveys to provide feedback on whether these notes were helpful or not (Kowalczyk, 2009).

The above-mentioned study is just one example of how information silos are maintained by a group of "keepers," perhaps both intentionally and unintentionally. Moves, such as the one described by Professor Delbanco and his colleagues, describe a way of breaking them down. With such actions, some physicians do perceive a loss of power—although others are keen to see the possible benefits. Battles over institutional silos and information silos can range from minor disagreements to all-out war.

In the coming chapter we will explore the nature of stakeholder conflicts. Before we move on, however, we want to extend our use of stakeholder theory by pointing to a couple of models and examples. To better explain the common structure management, the flow of information, and the exercise of power, we will return to the work of Professor Edward Freeman and his colleagues.

4.5 MANAGING FOR STAKEHOLDERS IN HEALTH CARE

In the book *Managing for Stakeholders*, Freeman and colleagues (2007) write of different types of "managerialism." They name a few major types of managerialism, one of which they describe pictorially in a two-dimensional pyramid (see Figure 4.2). This pyramid demonstrates the hierarchical nature with which more traditional firms prioritize their key stakeholders (Freeman, Harrison, & Wicks, 2007). In this model, the shareholders are the most important stakeholder group, followed by the corporate board, management, and the employers. We see in Figure 4.2 that other groups, such as the media and activists, may have some influence on corporate board operation, but they are not really prioritized into the structure. Also, the community and customers are equally unimportant in terms of their influence upon the company's functioning. Their input may be noted by the employees, but neither the management nor the corporate board would take an interest in putting the community's concerns first. As for the consumers, in this model, they may be noticed only when sales are falling.

Although it may seem as if this model is an arcane version of a corporation, Freeman and his colleagues (2007) suggest that this type of structure still exists.

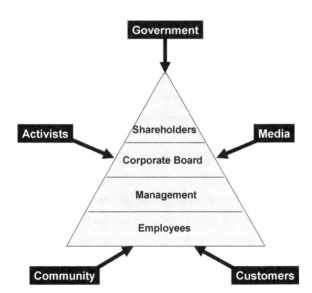

FIGURE 4.2 Freeman et al.'s managerial model: hierarchical view. From *Managing for stakeholders: Survival, reputation and success*, Fig 2.1, p.24 in Freeman, R. E., Harrison, J. S., & Wicks, A. C. Copyright 2007 by R. Edward Freeman, Jeffery S. Harrison, and Andrew C. Wicks. Adapted with Permission from Yale University Press.

Smaller, simpler versions of this pyramid diagram may also be present within the health care environment. The pyramid simply embodies a management style where the shareholders are the boss. All other stakeholders, including the customers, who in terms of health care may be the patients themselves, are seen as the inferiors.

A second model Freeman and his colleagues (2007) propose is one demonstrating the inwardly focused managerial view (Figure 4.3). This model portrays a style of management where there is attention focused inward at the shareholders. In this ecology, the management of the entity does not look for new opportunities such as diverse sources of growth and innovation outside the interests of the shareholders. In this model, there are grave trade-offs between satisfying the shareholders and satisfying the employees and customers.

There is no doubt that trade-offs among consumers, employees, and shareholders can result in disasters, especially in leaner times when customers are more selective and shareholders are more demanding. As Freeman and colleagues (2007) point out, in times of economic uncertainty, trade-offs result in unpredictable outcomes that are typically negative. In the above two models, the managerial style has made it difficult, if not impossible, for the entity to take advantage of information from different stakeholder groups. In a typical business scenario, this might mean that such a corporation, with a hierarchical or inwardly focused view, will eventually struggle to follow the customer and will come under fire from consumer groups. In a worst-case scenario, not being aware of other stakeholders could lead to a public relations nightmare with denunciations from activists, expository media reports, and legal repercussions, if government also gets involved. In the health care environment,

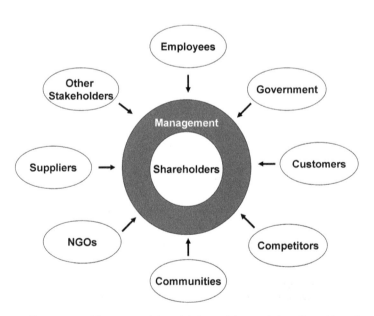

FIGURE 4.3 Freeman et al.'s managerial model: inward-focused view. From *Managing for stakeholders: Survival, reputation and success*, Fig 2.2, p.25 in Freeman, R. E., Harrison, J. S., & Wicks, A. C. Copyright 2007 by R. Edward Freeman, Jeffery S. Harrison, and Andrew C. Wicks. Adapted with Permission from Yale University Press.

poor understanding of other stakeholders can lead to all of the above, plus worse outcomes for patients.

Indeed, not being able to properly communicate a dangerous trend to physicians, such as the overuse of computed tomography (CT) scans, can have terrible consequences in terms of health outcomes and higher costs. As is described in Chapter 2, we now believe that a more intensive use of CT scans can mean a theoretically raised risk of radiation exposure in a patient population (Brenner & Hall, 2007). However, if one stakeholder group, such as the hospital management or a payer, cannot clearly understand the reasons behind why so many CT scans are prescribed, then these stakeholder (payers, doctors, consumers, management) may be unable to find the path to appropriate CT use. If physicians, payers, and the patient are in conflict over the appropriate use of CT scans, the patient may suffer in terms of lower-quality care. Certainly, as we outlined earlier, many physicians may resist clinical guidelines for myriad reasons, including a desire to maintain their current doctor-patient relationships, a fear of litigious patients, and conflicting interpretations of the literature (Mendelson & Carino, 2005; Studdert et al., 2005).

This could mean that pressure from the patients might guide a physician to prescribe a certain treatment or medication for fear of liability. Decisions made on this basis could influence the physician to emphasize defensive rather than preventative medicine. Defensive medicine has also been defined as "assurance practice" and is the behavior of ordering more tests, diagnostic procedures, and referrals for consultations with specialists. In a survey completed by more than 800 physicians, 93% said they had practiced defensive medicine. In that same survey, about 40% said they avoided caring for patients with complex problems—or patients they perceived as being likely to sue them (Studdert et al., 2005).

While defensive medicine means that patients will be consuming more in terms of health care dollars, the patients are getting less in terms of appropriate care. If we take Freeman et al.'s (2007) models and adapt them for analyzing problems in health care, we will soon see that it is not only "shareholders" who are prioritized over other stakeholders. The mistake we often see is that one stakeholder group will prioritize another group over everyone else. In certain instances, a private practice may focus entirely on thwarting litigious patients, to the detriment of their other stakeholders. Among large teaching hospitals, we may see some focused on keeping and attracting talented clinicians to the detriment of other stakeholders who hope to control Medicaid costs, for example. Among the large insurers, we may see some focused on satisfying their shareholders to the detriment of their ability to cover more patients, more procedures, and more preexisting conditions.

The point being made here is that many health care entities, regardless of their size, influence, and function, do not manage for the many stakeholders that they come into contact with on a daily basis. Because they do not manage for the many stakeholders that participate in health care in their immediate vicinity, they will find themselves coming into "stakeholder conflict." Freeman et al. (2007) used the expression "stakeholder conflict," but they did not define it to the extent that we will define it. We explore this concept in greater depth and detail alongside the concept of value in Chapter 5.

REFERENCES

Aetna. (2009). Aetna mission & values. Retrieved September 16, 2010, from http://www.aetna.com/about/aetna/ms/

Allen, S., & Bombardieri, M. (2008, November 16). A healthcare system badly out of balance. *Boston Globe*. Retrieved December 1, 2010, from http://www.boston.com/news/local/articles/2008/11/16/a_healthcare_system_badly_out_of_balance/

Allen, S., & Krasner, J. (2009, January 6). Tufts to break with Blue Cross: Hospitals take high-risk step over doctor pay. *Boston Globe*. Retrieved December 1, 2010, from http://www.boston.com/news/health/articles/2009/01/06/tufts_to_break_with_blue_cross/

Association of American Medical Colleges. (2009). AAMC thanks Obama administration for preventing payment cut to teaching hospitals. Retrieved September 17, 2009, from http://www.aamc.org/newsroom/pressrel/2009/090804.htm

Association of American Medical Colleges. (2010). Teaching hospitals. Retrieved July 16, 2010, from http://www.aamc.org/teachinghospitals.htm

Banner Health. (2009, July 8). Our nonprofit mission. Retrieved July 8, 2010, from http://www.bannerhealth.com/About+Us/Our+Nonprofit+Mission/_Our+Nonprofit+Mission.htm

Boudreau, K. J., & Lakhani, K. R. (2009). How to manage outside innovation: Should external innovators be organized in collaborative communities or competitive markets? The answer depends on three crucial issues. *MIT Sloan Managment Review, 50*, 69–76.

Brenner, D. J., & Hall, E. J. (2007). Computed tomography—an increasing source of radiation exposure. *New England Journal of Medicine, 357*(22), 2277–2284.

Center for Integration of Medicine and Innovative Technology. (2009). CIMIT consortium institutions. Retrieved September 14, 2009, from http://www.cimit.org/about-consortium.html

Centers for Medicare and Medicaid Services. (2009). Mission, vision & goals: Overview. Retrieved September 16, 2009, from http://www.cms.hhs.gov/MissionVisionGoals/

de Brantes, F., Gosfield, A. G., McGlynn, E., Rosenthal, M., & Levin-Scherz, J. (2006). Clinical practice guidelines for older patients with co-morbid diseases. *Journal of the American Medical Association, 295*(1), 34; author reply 34–35.

Duke University Health System. (2009). What is a teaching hospital? Retrieved September 12, 2009, from http://www.dukehealth.org/HealthLibrary/HealthArticles/teaching hospital

Freeman, R. E., Harrison, J. S., & Wicks, A. C. (2007). *Managing for stakeholders: Survival, reputation and success*. New Haven, CT: Yale University Press.

Garvin, D. A., & Roberto, M. A. (2002). *Paul Levy: Taking charge of the Beth Israel Deaconess Medical Center (A)*. Boston, MA: Harvard Business School Publishing.

Gilbert, S. J. (2008, September). The silo lives! Analyzing coordination and communication in multiunit companies. *HBS Working Knowledge*. Retrieved September 21, 2008, from http://hbswk.hbs.edu/item/6011.html

Kirch, D., Joshi, M., & Steuerle, C. E. (Speakers). (2009, August 20). *Medicare Spending*. Panel discussion presented at Fact vs. fiction: Key issues in health reform at the National Press Club, Washington, D.C. [Audio podcast]. Retrieved from http://www.healthaffairs.org/issue_briefings/2009_08_20_fact_vs_fiction/2009_08_20_fact_vs_fiction.php

Kleinbaum, A. M., Stuart, T. E., & Tushman, M. L. (2008). *Communication (and coordination?) in a modern, complex organization*. Unpublished manuscript.

Knox, R. (Writer). (2009). Doctors don't agree on letting patients see notes [radio feature story], *Your health*. USA: National Public Radio.

Kowalczyk, L. (2009, June 19). Patients to get a look at physicians' notes: Beth Israel study tests online access. *Boston Globe*. Retrieved December 1, 2010, from http://www.boston.com/news/local/massachusetts/articles/2009/06/19/patients_to_get_a_peek_at_physicians__notes/

McGlynn, E. A. (2003). An evidence-based national quality measurement and reporting system. *Med Care, 41*(1 Suppl), I8–15.

McGlynn, E. A., Kerr, E. A., Adams, J., Keesey, J., & Asch, S. M. (2003). Quality of health care for women: A demonstration of the quality assessment tools system. *Medical Care, 41*(5), 616–625.

Mendelson, D., & Carino, T. V. (2005). Evidence-based medicine in the United States—de rigueur or dream deferred? *Health Affairs (Millwood), 24*(1), 133–136.

Merriam-Webster Online. (2009). patient. Retrieved December 1, 2010, from http://www.merriam-webster.com/dictionary/patient?show=0&t=1291251396

Mitchell, R. K., Agle, B. R., & Wood, D. J. (1997). Toward a theory of stakeholder identification and salience: Defining the principle of who and what really counts. *Academy of Management Review, 22*(4), 853–886.

National Cancer Institute. (2010). NCI mission statement. Retrieved July 16, 2010, from http://www.cancer.gov/aboutnci/overview/mission

National Association of Urban Hospitals. (2009). *Urban safety-net hospitals and the American health care safety net*. Retrieved September 12, 2009, from http://www.nauh.org/docs/p2/Intro_NAUH_june09.pdf

NYU Langone Medical Center. (2009). About us. Retrieved September 22, 2009, from http://www.med.nyu.edu/about-us

Oxford Dictionaries Online. (2009). patient. Retrieved June 7, 2009, from http://www.askoxford.com/concise_oed/patient?view=uk

Pear, R. (2009, September 8). Data fuel regional fight on Medicare spending. *New York Times*, p. A12.

Quinlan, J. (2008, June 11). Revising the mission of Massachusetts General Hospital [Web log post]. Retrieved from Commonhealth blog at WBUR: http://archives.commonhealth.wbur.org/2008/06/11/revising-the-mission-of-massachusetts-general-hospital-by-joan-quinlan#more-499

Silber, J. H., Rosenbaum, P. R., Romano, P. S., Rosen, A. K., Wang, Y., Teng, Y., et al. (2009). Hospital teaching intensity, patient race, and surgical outcomes. *Archives of Surgery, 144*(2), 113–120; discussion 121.

Steinberg, E. P., & Luce, B. R. (2005). Evidence based? Caveat emptor! *Health Affairs (Millwood), 24*(1), 80–92.

Studdert, D. M., Mello, M. M., Sage, W. M., DesRoches, C. M., Peugh, J., Zapert, K., et al. (2005). Defensive medicine among high-risk specialist physicians in a volatile malpractice environment. *Journal of the American Medical Association, 293*(21), 2609–2617.

U.S. Department of Veterans Affairs. (2009). Locations. Retrieved September 12, 2009, from http://www2.va.gov/directory/guide/home.asp

Wertheimer, L. (Writer). (2009). Doctors on salary, one key to Mayo's success [radio broadcast]. *Health care*. USA: National Public Radio.

Wikipedia. (2009). Patient. Retrieved September 18, 2009, from http://en.wikipedia.org/wiki/Patient

5 Desperately Seeking Stakeholder Alignment: A Case Vignette

5.1 GOING TO WAR VERSUS SEEKING ALIGNMENT

There is one area of the health care debate that has increasingly been characterized with the rhetoric and verbiage of war: payment negotiations have evolved to become an area of vast complexity and strategic intrigue. There are no simple barters between hospitals, physicians, payers, and purchasers about payments for treatments and services in health care. These days reimbursements involve wrangling over very specific details concerning quality and treatment decisions. It is an understatement to say that these talks can be contentious and at times counterproductive; as we highlighted in Chapters 2 and 3, the crippling costs of care mean that an increasing number of people have either been priced out of health care altogether or settled for less than adequate insurance coverage. The Health Care and Education Reconciliation Act of 2010 was passed to modify this circumstance. While it is easy to see the pain that price inflation inflicts on patients and purchasers, all stakeholders, including payers, insurers, hospitals, physicians, and consumer-patients, struggle with rising costs. Often it might seem that the pressure to keep health care affordable falls squarely on employers, the government, hospitals, and medical group practices.

For the many stakeholders in health care, this signals that at least one stakeholder is going to lose out in terms of payments, due to the economic pinch that comes with trying to contain costs. It comes down to the old notion of "a dollar gained in your pocket translates into a dollar lost from my own pocket." Perhaps, then, it is unsurprising that there is plenty of rhetoric predicated upon the belief that changes implemented to curb health care spending will bring great pain to one or more battling groups of conflicted stakeholders. Evidence for these assumptions is everywhere, even among my colleagues who are trained to see both sides of the metaphorical coin.

A number of years ago, Harvard Business School Professor Regina Herzlinger wrote: "The U.S. health care system is in the midst of a ferocious war." She characterized the warring stakeholders as coming from four camps or, in her words, "armies . . . battling for control." Professor Herzlinger labeled these "armies" as "the health insurers, hospitals, government and the doctors." She also wrote that the individuals who are both the payers and the patients are the main losers, despite not even being immediate combatants in this war. According to Professor Herzlinger, the doctors also stand to lose a great deal. She argued that the physician group is the stakeholder most closely aligned with the patient-payer, and that physicians are the only other stakeholder with the patients' best interests at heart (Herzlinger, 2007).

We must ask ourselves if this is a totally fair characterization of the several stakeholders. Certainly, it is a perspective that favors the doctors, who are portrayed as a sort of casualty for targeted cuts in spending. Luckily, in recent years there has emerged a voice in the literature (and in practice) that points to the increasing need for true value to be a part of health payment negotiations. But what is meant by the word "value"? As individual consumers, we may use the word "value" all too loosely. We often say thoughtlessly, "Oh, that has good value!" when referring to Halloween decorations marked down on November 1, for example. We might find ourselves also saying this about a jumbo-sized tub of mayonnaise that we perceive as having more value per ounce than a regular jar. Many of us have been raised on the idea that buying more now for less money is good value.

When we look a little closer, the purchase of a giant tub of mayonnaise might not have been such a wise choice. Given that we do not need the giant tub for a massive egg salad to be served at a party, we have actually squandered other resources. After all, the tub of mayonnaise will sit in the refrigerator taking up precious space. In some cases its mere presence will encourage us to consume more than we need, possibly making us heavier. Also, by buying the huge tub we have tied up more of our monthly budget (our working capital) for food necessities on something that is perhaps, by all fair judgment, completely unnecessary. In the worst-case scenario, the tub will sit unfinished long after its expiration date, and the money we invested in buying it (although initially less per ounce) will be mostly wasted.

You might observe, too, that mayonnaise is not the healthiest foodstuff to be consuming in excess. Much like certain health care purchases, value is absent when there is overuse, underuse, or inappropriate use. Certainly, much of the potential value we might expect from appropriate health care is seen in these three fundamental problems—overuse (often to thwart litigious patients), underuse when it comes to the ideal course of management for chronic diseases, and inappropriate use when redundant tests are ordered, when physicians diverge widely from treatment guidelines, or patients abuse or mismanage their prescriptions or treatments. All these elements contribute to waste within health care, but this is not an exhaustive list; these are just a few examples. The last element, inappropriate use, is an area that is hard to define and harder still for stakeholders in health care to agree upon.

In Chapters 5, 6, and 7, we present three different case vignettes that touch on aspects of identifying and curbing waste. Often health care professionals pinpoint different areas of waste because they come from different areas of health care and bring to the table different perspectives regarding what actions, strategies, and behaviors are wasteful. What is one person's steak is another person's fat. It is far easier for a member of one stakeholder group to find fault with the actions of another group, rather than turn a critical eye to members of his or her own cohort. Before presenting these case vignettes, let us momentarily focus on defining value through the elimination of waste.

5.2 LEARNING ABOUT VALUE THROUGH THE ELIMINATION OF WASTE

The above digression about a large tub of mayonnaise shows that we must come up with a better definition for what we consider to be "value." When we talk about value, we must abandon the more-for-less paradigm which has been impressed upon us by Madison Avenue and perhaps a deeply engrained human sense of hoarding for leaner times. Fortunately, there is no lack of relevant literature on what connotes value; but only some literature is worth earnest review and reflection here. Bringing value to health care means that there is a constant promise to continually improve health outcomes through better prevention and treatment models. This also means improvement in our ability to catch a problem before it turns into a chronic disease, so we need better tools and the best use of the tools that allow for the diagnosis and prognosis of health issues.

There are a number of contemporary and historical methods to pursue continual improvement in a system. We start here with our discussion of value delivered through the elimination of waste, a philosophy that was, as we mentioned in Chapter 1, pioneered by Taiichi Ohno (Murman et al., 2002; Ohno, 1988). He saw the elimination of waste (*muda*), inconsistency (*mura*), and unreasonableness (*muri*) as the key to bringing more value to car manufacturing (Murman et al., 2002; Ohno, 1988). Mr. Ohno was also a proponent of asking all stakeholders to self-evaluate for areas of waste and wasteful habits (Ohno, 1988). The difficulty is that when anybody talks about the elimination of waste in health care, it very quickly sounds like grandstanding. Discussions of waste can easily deteriorate into finger-pointing episodes where one stakeholder is blamed for wasting another's money. However, the pointing game is destructive and dangerous. One entity may be able to align some stakeholders against others in the short term, but in the long run finger pointing is generally detrimental. An example of this would be when the U.S. House of Representatives Speaker Nancy Pelosi called health insurers "villains" in the summer of 2009, during the heat of the health care reform debate (Abelson, 2009).

Pelosi's charge was seen by many as counterproductive to the goal of reaching stakeholder alignment ahead of a push for health care reform. Moreover, talking about waste "in the health care system" is not at all productive. This is because a system itself, whether it is large or small, is not the generator of waste. Waste is generated from the everyday workings and the details of the interactions and transactions in the treatments and service exchanges conducted by the stakeholders that make up health care. It is not adequate to state that there is much duplication in billing and administrative practices. While this may be a truthful statement, it does not capture the waste in other stakeholders. The patient may also be wasteful in his or her behavior. This waste takes the form of noncompliance to prescribed medication, or a person's refusal to change a certain unhealthy lifestyle despite strong urging from clinicians. Perpetrators of waste can be completely unaware that their behavior, methodology, or processes are wasteful. And so, as often is the case, pinpointing waste is not difficult; it is the effort to change the wasteful behavior that presents the biggest challenge.

As we mentioned previously, there is great deal of variation in health costs and health outcomes among the many different types of hospitals, medical centers, specialists, and physician practices in the United States. Some of these differences can be characterized as regional, with wage discrepancies and building and rental costs figuring into the higher costs of care in the more urban, coastal settings (Pear, 2009). However, some variation in quality and cost of care may be found in the same town or city, or in two similar places, suggesting differing levels of efficiency. A series of pioneering studies published in 2003 looked closely at the differentials in Medicare spending and correlated them to the spending with health outcomes (Fisher, 2003; Fisher et al., 2003a, 2003b). The findings clearly showed that more spending does not guarantee a higher quality of care as measured by survivability, health outcomes, and even patient satisfaction in a cohort of Medicare patients with afflictions such as hip fractures, colorectal cancer, or myocardial infarction (Fisher et al., 2003b).

Another one of my Harvard colleagues, Dr. Atul Gawande, has emphasized the existence of pockets of greater value in health care throughout the United States (Gawande, 2009; Gawande, Berwick, Fisher, & McClellan, 2009). In a 2009 article, he and colleagues wrote: "[I]n studying communities all over America, not just a few unusual corners, we have found evidence that more effective, lower-cost care is possible." Dr. Gawande found these unique enclaves of low-cost, high-performing "medical communities" because they were outliers when he and his colleagues were trawling through the Medicaid and Medicare spending data. He also wrote a narrative about a high-cost medical community in Texas; despite the lavish amounts being spent on patients in that Texan town, the health outcomes were average, or even below par, when compared to outcomes achieved in similar, neighboring towns (Gawande, 2009). Dr. Gawande makes a suggestion that is practical and prescriptive: he and his colleagues ask that we study the success stories that exist—the "medical communities" that have sought to minimize waste. These are places run by people who have confronted high costs and slipping quality and found routes to improving quality while keeping costs under control, or even lowering costs. Indeed, these are the places that have sought to find true value in health care. Gawande and his colleagues have characterized them as the "positive outliers" among the average health care communities that provide care across the United States (Gawande et al., 2009).

With that said, we do not want to focus too much on the extraordinary outliers; instead we will look at the average range of issues that most stakeholders face on a daily basis. Stakeholders in health care, both large and small, face many separate and continual challenges related to delivering quality care for an affordable price.

Yet these challenges are similar in that they involve the seeking of consensus among other stakeholders. Perhaps the biggest challenge that I hear of is the difficulty in seeking alignment over issues that relate to improving health care through eliminating inefficiencies. There is a lot of talk about introducing higher efficiency among and within health care, but this rhetoric may not include a really rigorous identification of waste. Later we can look at models that help stakeholders think through a methodology that helps identify and eliminate waste.

At this juncture, we want to move onto the first of the three case vignettes presented in this book. These case vignettes offer a slice of life in a typical day of a number of health care stakeholders struggling to add value to health care. They are not studies of isolated success stories; instead they are ordinary and true-to-life representations of health care delivery in the United States. They are scenarios where stakeholders are struggling to find ways to improve health care quality and delivery while meeting the many demands to keep costs down or lower them further. In other words, we are not presenting cases about health care utopias or ivory towers within U.S. health care. These are real-life narratives about how change is already occurring in many small and large ways. In these narratives, you may find plenty of evidence of how difficult it is to align stakeholders to a common goal. A careful read of the vignettes may also reveal a sense of how alignment is always possible, especially when trust is established. Most importantly, I want to emphasize an argument that I made in earlier publications–that the return on investment from establishing trust can bring a windfall of opportunities for containing costs while maintaining or improving quality (Shore, 2005, 2007) So, without further delay, I move on to the first case vignette.[1]

5.3 THE WAR VETERAN

Thomas Jones[2] looked up from his Blackberry. He was talking about the stakeholders that he interacted with daily. They are the insurers, the employers, and the employee benefit consulting companies often enlisted to examine statistics in an attempt to characterize value by quantifying costs and performance of a hospital, a department, or a group of specialized physicians. As the chief negotiator at a large health system on the East Coast, he had heard just about every argument there is to make about lowering hospital reimbursements. His position in a system that encompasses a number of hospitals and care facilities speaks to his years of experience in the trenches of difficult, indeed contentious, payment negotiations. When we asked him to characterize the rapport between his health system and the stakeholders he interacts with on a daily basis, he said that each relationship is unique. As Mr. Jones

---

[1] This case vignette is the result of numerous interviews and communications carried out by phone, in person, and through e-mail correspondence.

[2] Names have been changed, and in all instances within the context of this case vignette and book "Thomas Jones" is used as a pseudonym to protect the interviewee's identity.

put it, the tone of the relationship varies greatly between different stakeholders depending on the details that dominate the negotiations. Some of these relationships are contentious, and some are more conciliatory. He also said that for him, it would be almost impossible to make general statements about any one of those relationships without knowing what the details of the relationship are. He put it this way:

Elements of the relationship have a lot to do with how prices are set, what they are set for, what are the conditions under which they are paid and not paid, and then what are the loopholes the insurers and the providers use in order to either maximize payment on the hospitals' side, or minimize payment on the insurers' side.

Mr. Jones paused and took a deep breath before reflecting on the meeting he had just attended. When we first spoke to him, he had just met with his peers—a national professional association of negotiators from various hospitals and health systems. At these meetings the association members swap stories, advice, and strategies. Over the years, Mr. Jones began to notice several trends. Importantly, it became clear to him that not all hospitals are likely to thrive or even survive. He says this is because there is great variation in how hospitals manage their costs and revenues and deal with managed care organizations. Some hospitals, he notes, face desperate financial straits despite having good clinical programs and a solid track record of performance.

The way Mr. Jones sees the situation is that a hospital's sustainability is closely linked to its ability to negotiate and enforce certain rates of reimbursements from its payers. He even sees large regional discrepancies that characterize hospital–payer relations when comparing the Southwest with the Northeast: "You would be surprised that the people in Iowa, Idaho, Texas are far more sophisticated then the New York hospital community." These differences, he explains, may be due to the fact that some Northeastern states, such as Massachusetts, New York, New Jersey, and Connecticut, had been controlled partly by "rate regulation" and "certificate of need approval for capital expenditures" in the past. This was a situation where certain prices were set and controlled by the government by linking commercial insurance payments to those made through Medicare and Medicaid (Fraser, 1995). Because of this legacy, according to Mr. Jones, many of those who worked for the hospitals lack the skills needed to drive reimbursement negotiations.

The people who grew up in the hospital business over the last couple of generations didn't really have any business acumen. They were financial analysts and accountants. Then when rates were deregulated payers swooped in and took advantage of everyone.

Mr. Jones added that, in his view, it has taken years for some of the hospitals in his region to build the expertise to better negotiate with the purchasers and payers. In a later conversation, via e-mail, he added that when hospitals do not get what they want they tend to blame the insurance companies. On the other hand, insurance executives often see hospitals as demanding and inefficient. Yet these stakeholders need each other, according to Mr. Jones:

> Hospitals continuously need more revenue and more patients; insurers continuously need more members, or sales to hold down their expenditures. A good long-term relationship [sic] is cognizant of each side's interests and each stakeholder tries to build these interests into their deals.

Interesting also is his take on how the mode of deciphering cost affects a hospital's or a payer's ability to influence negotiations.

5.4 "CLOUT" VERSUS "MARKET PRESENCE"

Hospitals may have different methodologies and ways to be reimbursed by payers. For example, they may be paid on a case basis, or they may charge by an average per diem and the type of bed, or by a combination of methods, and adjust from there. For some negotiators, certain methods are more preferable than others because they line up expectations between payers and hospitals in a more conciliatory manner. Mr. Jones claims that this is the case for the case-basis way his health system charges payers. The case basis may assume, for example, a seven-day hospital stay, but if the hospital releases the patient earlier the hospital may gain a higher margin for the case. Payers are also eager to have a patient released from the hospital as soon as possible because it may curtail the costs of more inpatient visits with doctors, as well as pharmaceutical costs. Limiting time spent as an inpatient may also limit the patient's exposure to infection.

Finding the kind of alignment where both a payer and a hospital are satisfied with the structure of an agreement is difficult to achieve. Mr. Jones says that payers and hospitals are at odds with one another over issues such as rate-setting methodology, price trend, case-mix methodology, length of contract, prior approval, denials and payment process of insurer, billing procedures, and carve-out services. The list goes on, as there are numerous potential points of contention. According to Jones, "It is very difficult to achieve a working relationship between a payor-provider [sic] that transcends a transactional conflict about pricing on a per-unit-of-service basis." The per-unit-of-service basis is a scenario where revenue is achieved by determining a unit price and the quantity of service units provided. Jones wrote in another communication:

> There are ways to achieve financial alignment such as risk or shared marketing, but the skills and the cultures necessary for the parties to establish a sustainable relationship are not present yet in most markets.

Mr. Jones explained that in a vast number of places, payment negotiations begin with a type of standoff. Thinking back to the meeting he had recently attended with other hospital negotiators, Mr. Jones had this to say:

Everyone I talked to west of Mississippi and south of Washington DC starts their negotiation by terminating contracts. They meet with everyone in their organization, and everyone in their organization, from the nurses down to the trustees knows what it means to fight with the payer.

Fights with payers do not have to take the shape of an all-out war, though. Much negotiation is carried out in a far more subtle and constructive manner. As we mentioned earlier, hospitals across the nation have diverse methodologies to quantify the services carried out on their premises. One might say that in the simplest of terms, hospital services are typically divided into "inpatient" and "outpatient," but this alone could be a point of great discussion during reimbursement negotiations. Inpatient admissions have traditionally been far more costly, as the patient is admitted to the hospital and may stay overnight. In recent years, however, there has been a substantial shift, as many treatments no longer require inpatient admissions, and a growing number of procedures—including surgeries—are performed as outpatient services. There are two main reasons for this shift, according to figures gathered in a 2009 report for the National Center for Health Statistics (Cullen, Hall, & Golosinskiy, 2009).

Ambulatory surgeries (commonly defined as surgical and nonsurgical procedures carried out on an outpatient service in a hospital or at a freestanding center) have increased because of technological advances and changes to reimbursements. During ambulatory surgery, patients are treated but not admitted to a hospital and typically go home once they have been treated. Medical advances, such as the widespread availability of better anesthesia, allow patients to regain consciousness quickly post-treatment and to experience fewer adverse side effects. Many surgeries have become minimally invasive, using techniques such as laparoscopy, endoscopy, and laser surgery, procedures that are far less risky than older, conventional surgery techniques (Cullen et al., 2009). All these facts add up to very positive advances for patients. As mentioned earlier, minimizing hospital stays also means patients are less likely to pick up nosocomial (hospital-acquired) infections that commonly lurk in medical facilities. The cost to the payer is also lower. Hospitals have used the trend to develop dedicated facilities that specialize in similar, nonrisky procedures. These centers are often referred to as ambulatory surgery centers (ASCs).

There is a downside as well: some patients may benefit from spending a night or two under the care and observation of the hospital staff, or they may learn from the staff how to better manage their chronic condition. The value in staying overnight is therefore difficult to measure, but generally speaking there has been a push from the payers' side to limit and curtail inpatient stays. Two academics writing in the late 1980s observed that changes to the Medicare program allowed for expanded coverage of ambulatory surgery, and that this alone may have contributed greatly to the explosive growth of ASCs and ambulatory surgeries. They also found that growth in ambulatory surgery was mostly additive, and did not take away from the rate of procedures performed on the inpatient side (Leader & Moon, 1989). This seems to still be true today, with the rate of inpatient procedures remaining relatively stable despite the continued growth in ambulatory surgeries (Cullen et al., 2009).

Many hospitals have capitalized on the growth of ambulatory services, perhaps by building or investing in ASCs. Yet, Mr. Jones explains, at times payers insist on an outpatient price for procedures that may require extended or overnight stays—in other words, inpatient services. One example is bariatric surgery, which might require the patient to stay on the hospital premises and be monitored. The payer may insist on reimbursing the outpatient fee, but instead of simply accepting this Mr. Jones says he may consider other options: "I don't know if there is alignment, but [negotiating] it is actually accommodating it. For example, I might say: *I'll take less on the inpatient, I may move that price of the $8,000 [treatment] down to $7,500 if you give me another five or six hundred on the outpatient service, for certain ambulatory surgeries.*" This type of bartering, says Jones, is not only commonplace but also the only way hospitals manage to stay in the black.

However, he also warned that advances in medical practice sometimes mean a change in the location and duration of a hospital service. As we see a shift from the inpatient to the outpatient setting, Jones says he sees that a number of procedures have shifted from hospital-based outpatient settings to community-based physician offices. He warns that it is all too easy to conclude that a service offered in a physician office may be cheaper, but this is not necessarily the case. "To say then that healthcare gets less expensive as it moves from the most intensive setting (hospital) to the least intensive setting (physicians office) is at best, an incomplete understanding," Mr. Jones explained in a written communication.

Another, more recent evolution in the way payers and hospitals do business is that payers may insist on tying payments to quality measures. This seems like a good idea—after all, patients, purchasers (such as employers), and insurers want a guarantee of quality health care. From the negotiators' side, however, this too may place hospitals in a financially precarious position. Mr. Jones contends that tying quality to payment is simply another way to lower reimbursements by cutting the reimbursement to "before" and "after" payments, which are not guaranteed. He puts it this way: "I don't fall for the flavor of the month ideas, because it is very hard to get paid on the back end when you need the cash on the front end." He added that for most hospitals—even high-performing hospitals—it is very hard to present evidence of meeting simple national standards. An example of a national standard is giving a heart attack patient an aspirin as soon as he or she comes through the door. But even this rule is surprisingly hard to enforce in practice. "It sounds bad, if I say, I don't want you to pay me for quality. I want you to pay me for my costs."

Mr. Jones explained that in his experience, hospitals are neither fiscally healthy nor sick because of their quality; instead, their financial situation really depends on how a hospital forges its contracts with its payers. "Hospitals that are doing really well, do so because they have good contracts, and hospitals that do poorly, do poorly because they have bad contracts." At this juncture we reached a discussion about market clout, a topic we have touched upon in earlier chapters in this volume. Some hospitals, particularly well-known teaching hospitals, may rely heavily on their reputation and size to attract patients. Simply put, if patients always have a preference for a particular hospital, then that hospital is able to secure higher reimbursements than its competitors.

It is unsurprising, then, that Mr. Jones and other negotiators dislike the phrase "clout," because it connotes only reputation and does not necessarily take into account the skills and market knowledge that Mr. Jones often talks about as the necessary survival tools in the world of reimbursement negotiations. The fact of the matter is that patients, to a certain extent, actively choose to use one hospital over another—especially in metropolitan areas where there is a higher density of medical facilities. As Mr. Jones puts it, he and others in his position like to refer to a hospital's "market presence" when talking about customer choice, and "business acumen" when referring to a hospital's ability to secure a favorable contract with a payer. These terms encompass more than simply the idea of "hospital reputation" with customers and "clout" with, say, insurers and purchasers. In a written communication, Mr. Jones said:

Very often price is neither a function of cost or quality. Price has a lot to do with reputation and program availability with physician preference for site of practice, and with the insurers [sic] ability to sell various products that enable the patients to access providers they like, or need, or are close to home, with as little hassle as possible and at the lowest possible out-of-pocket expense.

So far in this narrative about a hospital negotiator, we have kept things simple, referring to hospitals and payers. But in fact there are always many more stakeholders involved, although they may not be as vocal until a situation arises, like a hostile standoff between a hospital group and an insurer. Earlier in this chapter we said that Mr. Jones related stories about how some hospitals always start negotiations by ending contracts with insurers. This move, of course, can attract great public attention, with the insurer in question appearing somewhat demonized by the hospital in certain situations. Patients immediately get caught in the lurch, as a preferred hospital goes from being accessible to an out-of-network facility.

Unsurprisingly, when these types of standoffs take place, all the other stakeholders—local politicians, the news media, patient advocacy groups, consumer groups, nurses, and doctors—come forward and weigh in on the dispute. If a hospital plays its cards right, it may have public opinion on its side in such a fight—but that is not always the case. Some hospitals, despite having great market presence, may still not be as able to negotiate a contract with an insurer that is fiscally sustainable. Worse still is a situation in which public opinion turns against the hospital, in which case the hospital is forced to scramble to forge a contract with a payer. Perhaps in such a scenario they would have to accept far lower reimbursements than they budgeted, or contractual terms of payments that are difficult to meet. "Since both sides have a lot to lose, there is a strong incentive to reach compromise and consensus," Mr. Jones wrote in an e-mail. However, Mr. Jones also testified to the fact that not all the staff members in a hospital system are aware of the stakes:

Lots of times the hospitals do not know what they are fighting for. They don't know what they want. They don't know what is good for them. Half of what I do is try to explain to people, no, you don't really want to [sign] this. If you do that you would make less money.

From this narrative, our reader may deduce that a successful hospital must have both market presence and a highly skilled negotiator that can successfully convince payers of the hospital's budgetary needs going forward. But reading between the lines and thoughts of Mr. Jones, I hope you can detect something else. A successful negotiator is also very aware of the other stakeholders in the game and of the power they hold in any given situation. Some managers use stakeholder mapping as a saliency tool that allows them to fully realize the power and possible influence other parties have on any given decision or situation, before it reaches a contentious standoff. In the next section we look at just how stakeholder saliency mapping can steer strategic decision making.

5.5 REVISITING SALIENCY MODELING

Depending on where you sit, you have probably read this case vignette with a specific perspective. From experience, I can tell you that a room full of executive participants will make many different observations. It is through sharing these observations that they will glean information they might otherwise not have discovered. They will then reach a number of different conclusions. In this book, we want our readers to see themselves in other stakeholders' shoes. The purpose of reading a case study is not to reinforce a perspective or something that is already known to the reader; the purpose is to become slightly disoriented from a known reality.

A good case study does what good theory does. It does not force a reader into a single conclusion; rather, it opens up perspectives that were otherwise not apparent to the reader. In the classroom, we also use case studies to help focus debate. The purpose of this case vignette and the ones that will follow is twofold. We wish to encourage readers to see different view points, but also to focus inward—perhaps to notice one's own shortcomings, but in the wider sense to see how stakeholder theory can be useful, even crucial, in moving toward greater alignment. The subject matter in the case vignette may or may not speak to a handful of issues that are salient from your own work or stakeholder group within health care. However, it provides ample material to discuss saliency modeling, the subject matter of this section.

In Chapter 4 we introduced stakeholder saliency, only mentioning in passing the development of *saliency modeling* that some proponents of stakeholder theory have put forward. Here we briefly review stakeholder modeling, looking at how it has been used in the past. One of the most prominent stakeholder saliency models was proposed by Ronald K. Mitchell, Bradley R. Agle, and Donna J. Wood (1997). They took Freeman's theory and devised a way of managing multiple stakeholding parties through a system of evaluating each and every stakeholder's weight or influence in any given situation. This, they believed, was necessary because, while Freeman coined the phrase "The principle of who or what really counts" (Freeman, 1984), actually figuring out how to quantify who is influential and manage them accordingly is a complex task. As Mitchell and colleagues (1997) put it, managers must try to understand how different stakeholders hold differing types of power and influence in any given situation.

The authors came up with a system of classifying stakeholders into what they called different "quality classes of stakeholders" (see Figure 5.1). They looked at a stakeholder's power, urgency, and legitimacy to weigh the stakeholder's saliency to influence any given situation (Mitchell et al., 1997). Looking at Figure 5.1, we can see their model, which suggested roughly three basic classes of stakeholders. The "latent stakeholders" are defined as those that have little ability to influence a situation and possess only one out of the three important attributes (see areas 1, 2, and 3 in Figure 5.1). Areas 4, 5, and 6 represent stakeholders that have two attributes and are therefore classified as the "expectant stakeholders," as they are likely to expect and garner attention from a manager. Area 7, a place where the attributes of power, legitimacy, and urgency intersect, is inhabited by the "definitive stakeholders," the most influential stakeholders. Finally, area 8 represents the non-stakeholders.

I often ask students and workshop participants if they think stakeholder saliency modeling can be applied to the health care environment. Many agree that it is ideal for understanding stakeholders in health care. Certainly, many academics have thought it to be a good starting point in the past. In this chapter, where we have included a case vignette about a hospital negotiator, we can think back to some of the examples raised by Thomas Jones about his daily negotiations with payers. With a few more details about different payers, we could even chart and capture exactly where each stakeholder lies in the above saliency model.

Initially, it might be easy to conclude that all payers must have every attribute, including the power, legitimacy, and urgency to make them "expectant stakeholders," since they are major players in the delivery of health care. Yet, if we look closer, payers do hold different places: some are large and may represent a huge portion of

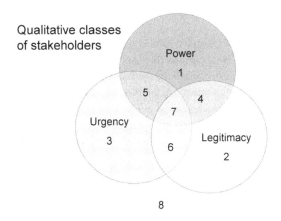

FIGURE 5.1 Stratifying stakeholders into classes. Adapted with permission from *The Academy of Management Review*, from "Toward a theory of stakeholder identification and salience: Defining the principle of who and what really counts," by R. K. Mitchell, B. R. Agle, & D. J. Wood, 1997, 22(4); permission conveyed through Copyright Clearance Center, Inc.

the hospital's patient-consumers, and therefore possess greater power than other payers. Some payers may be smaller but also have a greater urgency to renegotiate a contract. Depending on their relationship with a hospital network, this may make them weaker or more powerful in the eyes of a hospital negotiator.

The case vignette of the hospital negotiator is simple and has been stripped of all the insider strategies, which comprise the true back-and-forth that goes on between payers and hospitals. It is the perfect example for introducing stakeholder salience modeling. However, as the years have passed, I have found students and professionals asking increasingly complex questions about saliency modeling. Certainly, the relationships between stakeholders change over time, and may even change on a daily basis, depending on the microculture within a particular health care environment. The model in Figure 5.1 does not capture the fact that every relationship and situation may be in constant flux. Furthermore, it gives us no ideas as to how to come to alignment on issues of eliminating waste. We opened up this chapter with a discussion about value and how the word that connotes value does not carry the same meaning for every stakeholder. Therefore, in the next chapter I shift my attention not only to identifying salient stakeholders, but also to bringing salient stakeholders toward alignment on eliminating waste and creating value. We call this process the "onboarding" of salient stakeholders: it is a process by which salient stakeholders recognize and agree to address the inefficiencies of a particular aspect of health care provision or delivery.

REFERENCES

Abelson, R. (2009, August 5). For health insurers' lobbyist, good will is tested. *New York Times*, p. A1.

Cullen, K. A., Hall, M. J., & Golosinskiy, A. (2009). *Ambulatory surgery in the United States, 2006*. Atlanta, GA: Centers for Disease Control and Prevention/National Center for Health Statistics.

Fisher, E. S. (2003). Medical care—is more always better? *New England Journal of Medicine, 349*(17), 1665–1667.

Fisher, E. S., Wennberg, D. E., Stukel, T. A., Gottlieb, D. J., Lucas, F. L., & Pinder, E. L. (2003a). The implications of regional variations in Medicare spending. Part 1: The content, quality, and accessibility of care. *Annals of Internal Medicine, 138*(4), 273–287.

Fisher, E. S., Wennberg, D. E., Stukel, T. A., Gottlieb, D. J., Lucas, F. L., & Pinder, E. L. (2003b). The implications of regional variations in Medicare spending. Part 2: Health outcomes and satisfaction with care. *Annals of Internal Medicine, 138*(4), 288–298.

Fraser, I. (1995). Rate regulation as a policy tool: Lessons from New York State. *Health Care Financing Review, 16*(3), 151–175.

Freeman, E. R. (1984). *Strategic management: A stakeholder approach*. Boston: Pitman.

Gawande, A. (2009, June 1). The cost conundrum: What a Texas town can teach us about health care. *The New Yorker*, 36–44.

Gawande, A., Berwick, D., Fisher, E., & McClellan, M. (2009, August 13). 10 steps to better health care. *New York Times*, p. A27.

Herzlinger, R. (2007). *Who killed health care? America's $2 trillion medical problem—and the consumer-driven cure*. New York: McGraw-Hill.

Leader, S., & Moon, M. (1989). Medicare trends in ambulatory surgery. *Health Affairs (Millwood), 8*(1), 158–170.

Mitchell, R. K., Agle, B. R., & Wood, D. J. (1997). Toward a theory of stakeholder identification and salience: Defining the principle of who and what really counts. *Academy of Management Review, 22*(4), 853–886.

Murman, E., Allen, T., Bozdogan, K., Cutcher-Gershenfeld, J., McManus, H., Nightingale, D., et al. (2002). *Lean enterprise value: Insights from MIT's lean aerospace initiative.* New York: Palgrave.

Ohno, T. (1988). *Toyota production system: Beyond large-scale production.* New York: Productivity Press.

Pear, R. (2009, September 8). Data fuel regional fight on Medicare spending. *New York Times,* p. A12.

Shore, D. A. (2005). *The trust prescription for healthcare: Building your reputation with consumers.* Chicago, IL: Health Administration Press.

Shore, D. A. (Ed.). (2007). *The trust crisis in healthcare: Causes, consequences, and cures* (1st ed.). New York: Oxford University Press.

6 A New Framework for Studying Stakeholder Alignment

6.1 ON THE SUBJECT OF APPROPRIATENESS

In Chapter 5 we wrote primarily about the language of conflict in health care, and how a tone of war pervades health care delivery, including reimbursement negotiations. The language is part and parcel of a set of entrenched behaviors and assumed interests. In this chapter, we turn our attention to the language of alignment and how stakeholders occasionally attempt to find common ground despite their fundamentally different approaches to health care delivery. We lean heavily on the phrase "health care delivery" in this chapter because it is really the only phrase that captures the contribution of the different stakeholders and the confluence of different influences on the enterprise of providing care for patients.

Employers, insurers, hospitals, and physicians all influence health care delivery, along with many other salient stakeholder groups. Harvard Business School Professor Michael Porter and University of Virginia's Elisabeth Teisberg wrote about the "problematic" governance of physicians, especially when it comes to executing a more inclusive health delivery strategy in a facility like a hospital. The problem, as described by Porter and Teisberg (2006), is twofold. Firstly, some types of physicians may have stretched themselves thinly, perhaps treating a range of medical conditions (including some that fall outside their area of experience and expertise) out of financial necessity. Secondly, physicians, hospitals, and other providers are driven by areas of medicine that have "generous reimbursement levels."

In my own analysis, I ask students and professionals alike to reflect on not only the business proposition of providing care in the United States, but the business and professional risks of providing care to an increasingly litigious and difficult-to-please patient-consumer population. In other words, physicians, and even hospitals, can be profoundly influenced by the stakeholder group commonly referred to as "patients." No doubt that for many different types of providers and provider organizations, the benefits of practicing defensive medicine seem to far outweigh the (sometimes) theoretical hazards. Although many physicians might not openly reveal, some will admit (behind closed doors or among friends) that ordering unnecessary tests are a way of defending themselves against litigious patients, a behavior that is commonly seen as "defensive medicine" (Glabman, 2005; Studdert et al., 2005). A number of narratives from physicians interviewed on National Public Radio (NPR) capture these familiar sentiments well. Defensive medicine is not only a means of avoiding litigation; it is also a means of satisfying hard-to-please patient-consumers, who may have certain expectations about what constitutes good or even appropriate care (Glabman, 2005). When interviewed by radio reporter and host Melissa Block for NPR's *Morning Edition*, a family physician from New Mexico, Dr. Greg Darrow, had this to say:

There's an expectation for doctors employed by a large group to hit a *production target*... . Marketing, patient satisfaction, quarterly numbers, and all the business ends can intrude into the practice of medicine. (Block, 2009)

Dr. Darrow later added that physicians are not only pressured by their employers, or the partners that they work with, or their own practice's bottom line; patients also are increasingly pushy. He has found that patient-consumers often demand expensive imaging tests for minor injuries such as a twisted knee, which would typically resolve with adequate rest and ice (Block, 2009). With this and the multitude of other examples, it is possible to see that the focus in health care delivery today has evolved to proportion a higher priority to patient satisfaction over patient outcomes. Often, in various health care debates, patients are portrayed as a sort of innocent bystander. However, the market force that has almost euphemistically become know as "patient satisfaction" can be a greater influence than any other in certain situations. No doubt, it is health outcomes and survivability indicators that are a better measure for the performance of health care delivery, and not necessarily patient, or even doctor, satisfaction.

Chasing satisfaction on both the physician side and the patient side in the United States may have caused an interesting dichotomy in the delivery of health care. This point has not escaped the attention of insurers, who are particularly interested in curbing the use of tests and procedures that are inappropriate and possibly dangerous, and are invariably costly. Yet instituting strict guidelines or introducing cost sharing are often seen as having deleterious effects on care. Simply curbing costs by means of rationing health care and introducing greater cost-sharing as a disincentive to inappropriate use (i.e., having patients absorb a higher proportion of the cost through higher deductibles, higher co-pays, and less coverage for pharmaceuticals and certain tests and procedures) has been associated with hastening the poor management of chronic conditions (Solomon, Goldman, Joyce, & Escarce, 2009).

Some insurers, employers, and other purchasers are instead focusing efforts on promoting appropriate care (Glabman, 2005). However, these stakeholders alone are not well-equipped to institute change through unilateral measures that may otherwise be embraced by additional stakeholders. Instead, an approach that encompasses all stakeholders would be far more appropriate. We are back at our Gordian Knot analogy, where the dynamics of different forces not only act against one another but also are intricately and inextricably woven together. Stories and data about unnecessary intervention have stood at the forefront of the health care debate in recent years. Medical and public health policy journals are full of examples of how runaway interventional treatment has cost purchasers and payers not only great expense, but also their health (J. E. Wennberg, Bronner, Skinner, Fisher, & Goodman, 2009; Yasaitis, Fisher, Mackenzie, & Wasson, 2009). The larger theme of these critiques is that we spend a lot on care that does not help us, and could even harm us (Abelson, 2006; Brownlee, 2003; Gawande, Berwick, Fisher, & McClellan, 2009). But deciphering exactly what tests and procedures are necessary and beneficial in different instances is not an exact science, and oversight mechanisms are often complicated by purchasers and payers attempts to control costs.

Nevertheless, ways to ensure better care and better outcomes may exist. Much has been written about the benefits of active engagement between patients and physicians. Communication does lead to improved outcomes. Without a doubt, patient education about preventative care is a cornerstone of public health intervention strategy. Promotion of disease prevention through better awareness is a major tool used by health providers, consultancy groups, and government entities to cut expense while also promoting appropriate care. Even so, incomplete or improper implementation can render preventative care incapable of changing patient behavior most responsible for mortality and morbidity rates.

There have been some great historical successes with investing public money in preventative medicine. More recently, a number of health consulting firms have been offering an outcome-based approach to sizable purchasers of health care, promising not only a healthier, more productive workforce but also major cost-savings down the road. Health consultancy firm Pitney Bowes extols the merits of this approach, dubbing it "value-based benefits design" (Mahoney & Hom, 2006).

I have witnessed firsthand a huge growth in the use of consultancy firms by health insurers in recent years. One such consultancy firm, CareCore National, has garnered significant accolades for their ability to root out inappropriate care. As one of the firm's executives, Dr. Russell Amico, was quoted as saying in the *New York Times*, "We're seeing layering of tests on top of each other." He was suggesting that tests are often ordered together, unnecessarily, with more definitive tests occur alongside less useful and somewhat redundant tests (Berenson & Abelson, 2008). Yet many physicians will likely reject such a claim when shown a specific example in their area of expertise.

One area of medicine that has received much scrutiny lately is cardiac care. Contemporary computed tomography (CT) angiograms, for example, give physicians unprecedented moving images of the beating heart and its valves and arteries.

Even so, the proliferation and use of CT angiograms is not necessarily associated with better outcomes, or with high success rates for preventing cardiac events or improving cardiac care (Berenson & Abelson, 2008; Ladapo, Horwitz, Weinstein, Gazelle, & Cutler, 2009). A brief yet informative look at the different scenarios that influence the decision to use a CT scan can be found on the *New York Times* Web site (DeSantis, 2008), and we reprint it here in Figure 6.1. This diagram is not perfectly definitive; however, we believe it will help readers zero in on the issues discussed in the next case vignette and the literature review that follows it.

Figure 6.1 points to the crux of what many media outlets, including the *New York Times*, have recently questioned in the debate about "unnecessary" tests. The *New York Times* took a cynical view of the new CT technology, arguing that the CT angiogram may produce nice, compelling images of the heart but does not yield as much information as other, older tests. While this diagram highlights some important questions about CT angiograms as compared to other diagnostic tests, the newspaper oversimplifies the issue here. Firstly, it may be too early to know the full potential and insight that the latest CT scan technologies add to cardiac care. Secondly, we feel that decisions regarding appropriateness are far more complex than is portrayed in the examples here. But the fundamental question remains: "do new tests and treatments always, or nearly always, lead to better outcomes?

To better understand the complexity behind how diagnostic decisions are made, defended by specialists but questioned by purchasers, I thought it best to supply you with a case vignette. Certainly this next case vignette does not cover all aspects of cardiac care, guidelines, purchasers' concerns, or reimbursement negotiations. It does offer insight into how some clinical decisions and costs are viewed by stakeholder groups seeking alignment.

The case vignette is about a meeting of an insurance firm, a group of physicians specializing in cardiac care, and a hospital network that provides a highly specialized laboratory and clinic where the cardiologists practice medicine and carry out research. A close read of the vignette reveals that there are many other stakeholders that shape relationships and practices, even though they are not present at this meeting. There is, for example, a business consultancy group that the insurer has contracted but which is not represented at the meeting. There are competing cardiologists at other health systems and independent practices who indirectly determine the range of choices. There are testing centers that influence the cardiologists' work but which are mentioned only in passing. At this meeting, the most discussed stakeholder, who is noticeably excluded, is the patient.

This absence is certainly a logical one, given that the meeting is one in a series of physician payment negotiations. But it is also notable that the invisible hand of patient-consumer satisfaction may be driving much physician behavior. What patients expect greatly influences the measure of appropriate care. Yet, without having a seat at the table, the patient stakeholder group has some of its influences funneled through the actions and negotiating stances of purchasers. Their pull is exercised through another party, too, because generally speaking the insurers are representing employers, one of the major subsidizers of health care (along with the

The Unnecessary Medical Expense: A Case Study

One reason for high health care costs is that some expensive tests are frequently used even when they have not been proven to provide more useful information than older and cheaper tests. One example is the CT angiogram, a test that uses X-rays to produce detailed images of the heart and its arteries. Some other tests can provide more valuable information, sometimes at lesser cost. The chart below lays out both helpful and questionable uses of a CT angiogram, as described by Dr. Howard C. Herrmann, head of interventional cardiology at the Hospital of the University of Pennsylvania. The examples assume that each patient already had a simple electrocardiogram that produced normal results.

THE TESTS

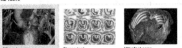

CT angiogram
The test, a series of X-rays, produces a composite picture of a beating heart and its main arteries. The scan can help rule out heart disease or show the formation of arterial plaque. If the patient has no plaque or blockages, testing can end. But if the patient has significant blockages, the doctor may proceed to other tests, including a stress test or a cardiac catheterization.
The CT angiogram test costs about $1,000 and involves significant radiation.

Stress test
There are different kinds of stress tests, all intended to produce a real-time chart or image of the heart as the patient exercises. Such tests can indicate areas of the heart that are not functioning normally, which might indicate blockages. The stress tests also provide the doctor with information like exercise capacity.
One common variety, the nuclear stress test, provides an image of the heart at work but involves significant radiation. It costs about $500.

Ultrafast scan
The test, also a series of X-rays, uses the same technology as the CT angiogram but does not require intravenous dye, as the CT scan does. The test, which produces a calcium score, looks for calcium deposits in the walls of the coronary arteries that indicate plaque. The scan may miss the soft plaque that would be seen in a CT angiogram or cardiac catheterization, but it can be used as a screening test.
The calcium score test costs a few hundred dollars and also involves radiation.

Cardiac catheterization
This test will determine definitively if the patient has heart disease, but the test is invasive. A catheter is inserted through the groin and threaded through blood vessels up to the heart. If, during testing, the doctor finds a significant blockage, the doctor can immediately treat the blockage with a stent — a mesh metal tube that props open the artery.
The catheterization might cost several thousand dollars, while a stenting procedure might cost an additional $7,500 or more. But in almost all cases, this test would be paid for by medical insurance.

ASSESSING CANDIDATES FOR A CT ANGIOGRAM

	Patient A	Patient B	Patient C	Patient D
	Male, 40 years old Low risk factors for heart disease Chest pain	Male, 60 years old High risk factors Chest pain	Female, 37 years old High risk factors No chest pain	Female, 55 years old Intermediate risk No chest pain
	Patient A comes into the emergency room complaining of chest pain. The patient has a history of heartburn and sometimes uses antacids for relief. The patient has high blood pressure but no other risk factors.	Patient B goes to a cardiologist complaining of chest pain. The patient has several severe risk factors associated with heart disease. He smokes, has a family history of heart disease and has high cholesterol.	Patient C goes to a cardiologist for a routine examination. Her mother, who died prematurely of heart disease in her late 40s, the patient once smoked and has mildly elevated cholesterol. She exercises regularly.	Patient D goes to a cardiologist because she has both high cholesterol and high blood pressure and is very worried about her risk of heart disease. She would like to decrease her risk by beginning an exercise program.
	Good candidate Patient A may or may not have a heart problem. The goal will be to quickly and definitively rule out heart disease as the cause of his chest pain. White observation and a stress test would require the patient to stay six to nine hours, a CT angiogram can be done quickly. If the test does not show signs of heart disease, the patient can immediately leave the emergency room. If the CT angiogram does indicate heart disease, the patient would stay for further tests.	**Poor candidate** The CT angiogram can help doctors definitively rule out heart disease. But even if a doctor does find significant blockage with the CT scan, there will need to be additional testing. In this case the patient's risk factors, combined with chest pain, make it likely that the doctor will find some kind of heart disease with the CT scan. So it makes sense to bypass this step and go directly to a stress test or a cardiac catheterization.	**Borderline candidate** Because of her family history, the patient will probably eventually be treated for her cholesterol with a statin drug. The CT angiogram would help screen the patient for early plaque deposits. If the test shows no sign of heart disease, the doctor might encourage dietary control of the cholesterol before starting her on a lifelong drug. But the CT scan is expensive, and an ultrafast scan would be adequate as a screening test in a young person. The ultrafast scan may also involve less radiation, which affects women more than men.	**Poor candidate** Patient D does not have any symptoms of heart disease and is unlikely to have severe coronary artery blockages. The CT angiogram would help discover any hidden arterial plaque, which might not warrant any treatment. But a stress test could also let the doctor know if the patient had heart disease — while also providing information about how well the patient's heart functions under stress.

Source: Dr. Howard Herrmann

government/taxpayers), as well as themselves. Even though this meeting is ultimately about reimbursements that are linked to physician services, it touches on a number of issues regarding decision making and care delivery, specifically in the area of appropriate imaging for cardiac patients.

As you read this case vignette, it is worth noting how stakeholders as diverse as physicians and insurers all seek to provide better value for the patients, yet they have strikingly different approaches. These approaches encompass their own strategic business needs as well as the patients' interests. Indeed, as one student of stakeholder theory wrote, it is the relationships governing stakeholders that are both "complex and dynamic" (Grossi, 2003). In his thesis, submitted for a Masters of Science and Engineering Management at the Massachusetts Institute of Technology, Ignacio Grossi (2003) integrates important concepts and tools to analyze stakeholder relationship and saliency. He proffers a systems approach to understanding how stakeholders are structured as a means of first understanding the dynamics of how these stakeholders can work together. Grossi developed a classification to help characterize the relationship between stakeholders. He also proposes better ways to create value between those very same stakeholders. We will illustrate some of Grossi's ideas toward the end of this chapter, after we have had a chance to unpack the many components of the case vignette.

The development of metrics to analyze stakeholder relationships has not been as succinctly developed as we might hope. To use these metrics, Grossi (2003) makes a number of assumptions. In at least one instance he assumes, for the purpose of modeling, that "relationships between stakeholders are bidirectional and balanced." In another variation of his DSM, he is able to account for asymmetries, or, as he puts it, "particular characteristic[s] of the relationships between stakeholders." Understanding the clustering and nature of stakeholder relationships with fine accuracy is not easily achieved, even when using specialized tools. With these shortcomings in mind, we still encourage the use of tools that facilitate a deeper understanding and foster a great deal of group discussion. Importantly, we want to stress the fact that analytical tools are only successful if the data used are accurate. In fact, we affectionately refer to the phenomenon of making decisions on bad data as "GIGO," or garbage-in-garbage-out. It is important to not blame the tools while understanding that in some cases bad decisions are predicated on bad data.

FIGURE 6.1 A *New York Times* case study. Source: DeSantis, A. (2008, June 29). The unnecessary expense: A case study. *New York Times*. Available at http://www.nytimes.com/imagepages/2008/06/29/business/29scan.graph1.web.html ©June 28, 2008 The New York Times All rights reserved. Used by permission and protected by the Copyright Laws of the United States. The printing, copying, redistribution or retransmission of the Material without express written permission is prohibited.

We should make one last caveat before delving into the details of the meeting featuring the insurer, the cardiac specialists, and representatives of the hospital network. In order to accurately capture the true nature of a stakeholder relationship, a great amount of human knowledge is needed. Relationships are moving targets, and so it is possible to see only a snapshot of a relationship when discussing stakeholder alignment. As we will see in later sections of this chapter and book, before the possibility of value creation arises, stakeholder alignment is an absolute necessity. This alignment is only possible after the different parties take the time to fully appreciate the shifting nature of their relationships. It is with these thoughts that we continue on to our next case vignette.

We revisit Thomas Jones, the chief negotiator for the large East Coast health system we mentioned in the Chapter 5, as he oversees contractual relationships of mostly third-party payers. In this case vignette he is hosting one of a series of talks regarding reimbursements for cardiac specialists who work in his network. Within a hospital system, the many community-based physicians who work on the premises establish their own contracts with payers independent of the hospital itself. Yet at times, Mr. Jones explained, this can lead to tension between the hospital and the visiting doctors: "If the doctor is working in one of our facilities and is self-employed, or employed by a group that we don't own or control, I can not set the price." The doctor, however, may expect that his or her reimbursement is contingent on the hospital's prenegotiated price. This is a problem, says Mr. Jones, because the expectations of the patients are far from being aligned with the hospital, the physicians, or the payers' expectations. What they want regarding who treats them, where they get treated, and how they get treated often confounds the delicate dividing lines among the provider groups. Often, it is this lack of transparency that may be at the heart of the distrust and occasional conflict between stakeholders.

Another source of conflict according to Mr. Jones lies in the process of creating contracts between insurers and hospitals. A hospital negotiates reimbursement rates without including physicians who are not directly employed by the hospital. This exclusion may exist despite the fact that the nonemployed physician works on hospital grounds. In contrast, employed physicians often work side by side with community, nonemployed physicians who have different relationships with the payers and at times are treating the same patients. The employed physicians are represented by the hospital and the contract or arrangement of the payers. Mr. Jones notes that this is a possible area of tension and misalignment: "Some of the physicians in the community may be getting paid more than some of the physicians that work at the hospital, while some get less. No one really knows," Jones said in a follow-up phone conversation. He explained that because all payment schedules are proprietary and confidential, no one is really sure how anyone else is getting paid, or whether a comparison would show reimbursement rates to be higher, the same, or lower.

When it comes to negotiating physician reimbursement, insurers have a vested interest in evaluating physician performance. They may focus their negotiations on indicators that try to characterize or measure efficient care. In recent years, one common measure involves whether physicians and other clinical staff are sticking to "appropriateness criteria" when ordering tests. In earlier chapters, we looked at how rapid spending paralleled a rise in imaging across the United States, and how there are large regional variations in ordering tests (Smith-Bindman, Miglioretti, & Larson, 2008; U.S. Government Accountability Office [GAO], 2008;

D. E. Wennberg & Wennberg, 2003). Physicians defend their decisions by relating them to the circumstances in which they order diagnostic tests. The poor quality of a test, or the report generated from the test, and the need for further clarification are often cited by physicians as reasons to repeat or reorder tests. In this light, physicians argue that measures curtailing their ability to order a diagnostic test comprise a blatant interference with physician autonomy.

The discussion outlined in the following paragraphs is between cardiac specialists and researchers who are employed within this particular health system and are therefore considered to be part of the system's core staff. The physicians, the hospital administrators, and the insurer are the three major players in this negotiation. As in our last case vignette, all the names of people and organizations have been changed here.[1]

6.2 THE MEETING

On a rainy summer day in 2009, Mr. Jones hosted high-level talks between his health system's cardiac specialists and a major insurer. The agenda outlined a number of presentations; among them was a PowerPoint presentation from the insurer introducing new performance criteria and programs, followed by a presentation by one of the health system's cardiac specialists summarizing findings from the health system's own patient population. Time was also set aside to discuss a series of studies comparing guidelines of appropriateness criteria for cardiac testing. First to present was Dr. Peter Morrow, a medical director at Bigtoe Insurance. He introduced results from a cardiac imaging program intended to curtail inappropriate testing. The goal of this program, explained Dr. Morrow, is to try to maintain or improve quality for patients. He maintained that Bigtoe Insurance is looking at clinical performance in terms of measurable cardiac outcomes. He also stated that a major goal is to try to maintain satisfaction among physicians and patients while eliminating inappropriate testing. Dr. Morrow reported that the insurer's approach to quality is to have heart specialists undergo precertification initiatives. For the health system, these initiatives imply that their cardiac specialists may need to take exams in order to prove a certain level of competence.

This program was not entirely novel. Bigtoe Insurance had introduced precertification requirements for nuclear stress testing, CT cardiography, and magnetic resonance imaging (MRI) in the past. But now they were also proposing to expand the program to encompass precertification for physicians ordering echocardiography, stress echocardiography, and diagnostic left heart catheterization. Dr. Morrow explained that the rationale behind the move was to utilize new criteria developed by the American College of Cardiology (ACC) and the Cardiology Foundation. He then posited that recent literature indicates that anywhere between 11% and 22% of testing ordered by physicians may be inappropriate, a percentage considered both too high and wasteful. To address this, Dr. Morrow reported that the insurer had

---

[1] The names used for Mr. Thomas Jones and for Drs. Peter Morrow, Angelo DiNardo, Conrad Shultz, Carl Patel, and Janet Dodd are all pseudonyms used to obscure the identity of case study participants. "Bigtoe Insurance" and "Balloon Consulting" are also pseudonyms for actual insurers and consultancies.

started to collaborate with the ACC to craft a proposal that would address inappropriate echocardiography use, particularly the repeat echocardiography ordered for patients within one year of initial testing. In summary, Bigtoe Insurance was delicately trying to introduce a new protocol whereby they could identify a group of physicians as "high-performing" cardiologists within Mr. Jones' health system. Those physicians labeled as being "high-performing" would not have the additional burden of going through a precertification process.

Next, Dr. Morrow detailed some of the criteria of how and under what circumstances Bigtoe Insurance identifies doctors and laboratories that meet their basic quality criteria. First, the doctors would have to be participating with Bigtoe Insurance already. Additionally, the laboratory where the echocardiology occurred would have to be credentialed under a recognized national accreditation program. He also mentioned that the practicing doctors needed to agree with the appropriateness criteria that had already been developed with the ACC, and if they were not going to be subject to precertification they would have to use some other method to justify the appropriateness of the echocardiogram that they were ordering. Individuals selected at higher-performing centers would not have to register the echocardiograms, but they would be asked to voluntarily enhance data collection and participate in a long-term study examining decisions to repeat any echocardiograms. Dr. Morrow contended that such data would allow the insurer and the ACC to better analyze all the usage patterns related to echocardiography.

In response to this presentation, the hospital's leading physicians articulated a number of questions and comments. First to speak was an "in-house" specialist, Dr. Angelo DiNardo, who wondered just how objectively the insurer, or a consultant to the insurer, could conduct the precertification process. Dr. DiNardo spearheads some major quality- and process-improvement programs and manages an institute that conducts cutting-edge research within the health system. His colleague, Dr. Conrad Shultz, who oversees cardiovascular services for facilities across the entire health system, acknowledged that Bigtoe Insurance's program was going in the right direction. He even mentioned that the program should encompass the staff interpreting the echo, adding that those qualified to do so were already subject to a rigorous fellowship program and a series of exams. He offered that Bigtoe Insurance could utilize the results from such a fellowship program.

To that point, Dr. Morrow said that there had been significant discussion between the insurer and the ACC, since the insurer had originally proposed a panel of board-certified "interpreters" that would assist in deciding which doctors may bypass the program altogether. Expanding on this point, Dr. Morrow's colleague Dr. Carl Patel explained that Bigtoe Insurance had partnered with health consultancy firm Balloon Consulting to generate reports on physician performance as far as appropriateness criteria is concerned. Mr. Jones interjected that Balloon Consulting had been the recipient of criticism for not giving adequate and transparent feedback to explain their methods, data evaluation, and communication with physicians. To this point, Dr. Patel emphasized that in setting up the program, Bigtoe hoped to instill a sense of trust among the doctors who enrolled. However, it became clear that the specialists at the table were not especially comfortable with the details of the new program.

Dr. Conrad Shultz took a moment to relay an anecdote about how he was denied a test on a patient, despite having a legitimate reason to order the test. He suggested that he and his cardiology colleagues in the health network already faced difficulties in reordering necessary tests, and he feared that retesting was often disallowed by an insurer for arbitrary reasons:

I had a patient that had a dissecting aneurism of the aorta fix, and an aortic valve replacement that I've been following for several years. The last echo I had on her was more than two years ago, and I decided to get an echo to see if the aorta was expanding. And, unfortunately, six months ago, her internist sent her somewhere to get an echo. And that echo, I had the report, it described a normal aortic valve—not even a prosthetic valve! So, how could I possibly rely on the information? Balloon Consulting denied the echo because she had one six months ago, so what recourse [do I have] to that?

In response to this story, Dr. Patel commented that the program Bigtoe was introducing was intended not to question the decisions made by every doctor, but to figure out which doctors should be designated "high-performing." He explained further:

In the bypass program we proposed no denials of anything, they [physicians] would tell us why they are getting an echo, and they would tell us the other echo doesn't appear to be accurate. That would appear to be a legitimate reason to say: *okay that's why you're getting another echo.*

Dr. Patel went on to say that Bigtoe Insurance hopefully satisfied the concerns of the ACC by making the transparency of their own appropriateness guidelines evident to all practicing cardiologists. He said that the insurer had worked out specific algorithms surrounding echocardiology, stress echocardiology, and the diagnostic catheterization certification program. At the time of the meeting, Bigtoe Insurance was engaged in ongoing discussions with the ACC to formalize data sharing, particularly on echocardiology. Mr. Jones commented that Bigtoe Insurance should be commended for taking the time and effort to explain their methods to specialist staff within his health system, adding that most insurers were not as forward-thinking. He then handed the floor over to one of his health system's cardiologists, Dr. Janet Dodd, who was presenting some of her team's own data.

Dr. Dodd, who is in charge of nuclear cardiology at one of the health system's specialty hospitals, started off her presentation by handing out a document comparing appropriateness criteria proposed by Bigtoe Insurance with that put forward by the ACC. She stated that the most recent version of the ACC's appropriateness criteria was published on May 18, 2009, and that it had been expanded recently to guide the use of nuclear imaging. She then highlighted a study that supported her concerns about the lack of overlap of the appropriateness criteria proposed by the ACC with the appropriateness criteria being adopted by Bigtoe Insurance.

I just told you the number of criteria the initial document analyzed here honed in on 52 [guidelines].... Current criteria will profile 66 [guidelines]. The overlap between those, and the original 50, and Bigtoe Insurance's [criteria] stands at 27 [guidelines]. And if you read those carefully, if you take, for example, the first one—you will see that not only the wording, the language, [and] the profile is different, but the whole approach and premise is different. Why is that the case?

Dr. Dodd also cited a memo written by Dr. William Van Decker of the American Society of Nuclear Cardiology (ASNC) to the U.S. Senate Finance Committee on the topic of health reform (Decker, 2009). In Box 6.1, you can see an excerpt from this memo, which comprises mainly feedback to early government proposals for health care reform involving imaging utilization. In the memo, Dr. Decker, the chair for the ASNC Government Relations Committee, makes it clear that the ASNC is opposed to mandatory lab accreditation and the declaration of appropriateness criteria regarding imaging. Dr. Dodd said that while these words seem "harsh," she believes the memo really does reflect the sentiments of most practicing cardiovascular physicians. She said this is the case because, in many ways, cardiologists see guidelines, particularly those laid out by insurers, as arbitrary. She argued that the Bigtoe guidelines were not something that practicing physicians could abide because the specialists believed the criteria failed to specifically include the multitude of clinical situations that require cardiologists to reorder tests.

Dr. Dodd then presented research she and her colleagues had conducted on appropriateness criteria and patient outcomes. She highlighted different studies

---

Box 6.1 The Physicians' Perspective

[The American Society of Nuclear Cardiology] ASNC was extremely pleased to see that the Senate Finance Committee is looking at alternatives other than radiology benefit managers (RBMs) as it looks to ensure appropriate imaging. As a physician organization, our experience with RBMs has been abysmal, and we are strongly opposed to an RBM mandate. RBM guidelines favor one imaging modality over another regardless of physician judgment, clinical factors and appropriate patient care. RBM guidelines are incongruent with current literature and imaging guidelines published by medical journals and medical specialties. The practice parameters created by RBMs do not involve direct input from actively practicing local physicians or relevant physician organizations prior to endorsement, and the RBM guidelines do not include rationales used to set their practice parameters. Their guidelines are usually based on initial cost containment only (indeed their own revenue stream is based on percent cost saved only) and do not reflect what is best for the patient or what downstream utilization and quality outcomes may be obtained.

Source: Van Decker, W. (2009, May 15). *Regarding the Senate Finance Committee's Health Reform Policy Options: Transforming the Health Care Delivery System: Proposals to Improve Patient Care and Reduce Health Care Costs* [Open Letter]. Retrieved June 19, 2009, from American Society of Nuclear Cardiology website: http://www.asnc.org/

(some unpublished) and gathered data with her colleagues on whether patients classified as inappropriate were in fact not deserving of the medical evaluations garnered through various imaging tests. She said that many of her findings were in line with published results from the Mayo Clinic. "An appropriateness criterion is a tool," she cautioned. "You want to make sure that a tool is clinically relevant." Dr. Dodd based her analysis on data pulled from her patient population. It showed that patients who had undergone tests deemed inappropriate by existing guidelines did have the lowest cardiac event rate. However, a small percentage of this population did experience a cardiac event shortly after being ruled as an inappropriate candidate for testing.

Inappropriate patients had the lowest event rate, it was a 2.4%, and certain patients came in the middle at a 7% [event rate]. So, as a practicing cardiologist, anything that exceeds 2% for us is a significant event rate. [The] 2.4% [event rate] is essentially our ground floor, and anything that gets above that is a serious event rate.

Dr. Dodd was making this point to demonstrate that she and her colleagues were not comfortable with seeing a higher percentage of patients labeled as inappropriate patients for testing. The 2% that would experience a later cardiac event was too much to accept. To this point, Dr. Shultz added his interpretation of the findings. He said that the kind of patient that he and his colleagues attract to their laboratory (which is also integrated into the health system) is very different from the patients seen by someone in a private practice. He maintained that a lot of patients are put through prescreening before they are seen by his staff, so they come in with known heart problems. He added that applying "blanket criteria" across a broad spectrum of patients (e.g., those who have already been prescreened versus those being seen for the first time) is, in his eyes, dangerous. Like Dr. Dodd, Dr. Shultz fears that people labeled as inappropriate by guidelines, or those denied coverage, may very well be good candidates for screening. Dr. Dodd added that her team was still investigating the reasons why appropriateness criteria were not sensitive enough to pick up patients who would otherwise be deemed appropriate by a specialist, or a patient who may go on to have a cardiac event despite having been ruled as inappropriate for certain screening tests.

As the specialists made their case for not being strictly tied to criteria that might curtail their use of screening tests, Mr. Jones, the hospital's negotiator, was intent on highlighting the research his hospital was able to produce. He summarized this to the insurer in a comment he made as Dr. Janet Dodd finished her presentation:

What I think what we are trying to do is, [we are] trying to propose a way of our doing business in this area with you, if you are open to it... there is an enormous amount of content and research and depth in our organization. It's to show you that we can control inappropriate use of this kind of testing.

Mr. Jones concluded his argument by reporting that he was proposing his health system's doctors and specialists should self-manage as far as appropriateness criteria were concerned, while keeping Bigtoe Insurance in the loop as far as data gathering on physician performance was concerned. He added that self-managing appropriateness criteria would allow the hospital system to attract more specialized doctors. Before wrapping up the meeting with some final comments, Mr. Jones did take a moment to digress on the topic of health consultants that regularly advise and inform insurers about projected health outcomes and performance as far as appropriateness criteria are concerned: "The consultants come in and they have very bad data . . . and they do not have the vested interests of the patients in mind." Mr. Jones made these comments perhaps as a cautionary note to Bigtoe to not rely too heavily on data gathered by Balloon Consulting.

Mr. Jones proposed several new programs and price-related negotiation tactics aimed at pending renewals of various contract deals with the insurer. He spoke of how his health system had sought to bring more doctors on board, and how it was reducing prices and adding wellness programs for patient-customers (and the employers of patient-customers) hoping to engage in more preventative care. To these comments, a representative of the insurer asserted that Bigtoe Insurance and the health system did indeed share a number of "goals" and "common ground." Shortly thereafter, the meeting ended with a promise to continue talks on different program proposals to be discussed among special task forces consisting of the insurer, the physicians, and hospital administrators.

6.3 A "STRESS TEST" FOR RECOGNIZING POTENTIAL ALIGNMENT

This case vignette is a moment in the life of several real health care stakeholders. The situation is a familiar one and is easily generalized for a wider understanding of stakeholder discussion. One of my graduate students summarized the literature that relates heavily to the above case vignette quite succinctly. We can distill the situation down to the bare bones of the literature that best summarizes the conflicts of interest these types of stakeholders face regularly. The following synopsis captures the concerns of the different stakeholders well; it also makes some assumptions that not everyone may agree with. This is simply one way of summarizing the stakeholders' perspectives; it is not the only way. We use this summary because it relates to current literature. My colleagues and I have since adapted it to use in a stakeholder role-play exercise that complements the case vignette.

Disease of the heart is said to be the leading cause of death in the United States (Heron et al., 2009). Recent advances in technology, both old and new, have contributed to the cost of care of cardiac patients. Tests that make use of echocardiology, cardiac CT, myocardial perfusion imaging, and cardiac MRI have shown varying degrees of accuracy in diagnosis and have therefore prompted questions about how and when these tests are used, what other tests they are used in conjunction with, and how they are ordered and interpreted (Hendel, 2008). Insurers and purchasers worry about the rising costs of newer, more expensive diagnostic tests (Glabman, 2005). They are also concerned that some tests may be duplicated or redundant when ordered indiscriminately, and that quality controls may be low among some imaging centers (Glabman, 2005; Seidel & Nash, 2004). More-recent literature has highlighted the theoretical effect of repeated and high exposure to radiation, and the possibility of follow-up procedures that may encourage unnecessary therapeutic interventions (Brenner & Hall, 2007). More generally, researchers have begun to focus attention on how intensive medicine may add little health benefit or even detract from the patients' health while adding great expense to care (Fisher, 2003; Fisher, Goodman, Skinner, & Bronner, 2009; Fisher et al., 2003a, 2003b).

Separately, and most alarmingly, the news media has picked up on pockets of cardiologists that demonstrate unusual interventionist trends and decision patterns, which stray from evidence-based medicine. In some of the worst-case scenarios, a handful of cardiologists demonstrating unusually extreme trends in practicing a high number of interventionist procedures have been investigated, sued, or even arrested by federal authorities. In one well-publicized case, a Louisiana doctor was charged with defrauding Medicare after having been accused of performing unnecessary procedures (Abelson, 2006).

Even when obvious fraud is not suspected, the news media has not let recent scholarly findings go unnoticed. Negative press is damaging not only to the specialists in question, but also to the hospitals where they practice, as well as to the field of cardiology as a whole. Patient–provider trust may be damaged or, worse still, irrevocably eroded. For example, the *New York Times* ran an article describing a group of Ohio cardiologists that appeared to perform angioplasties at four times the rate of the national average (Abelson, 2006). The information came to light following reports published by the Dartmouth Institute for Health Policy and Clinical Practice (2009). In recent years, the Institute's oft-quoted reports have been referred to simply as the "Dartmouth Data" and have highlighted the eye-opening discrepancies in trends of care across the United States. The Dartmouth Data tease apart the reasons behind obvious differences in the patterns of care and have recently zeroed in on what has been termed as differences in "local ecology of health care" and the "social norms" among physicians as two of the leading factors guiding decisions in care (Fisher et al., 2009).

It is practically indisputable that the practice of cardiology is one of the most lucrative areas for hospitals and networks of providers and physicians. Investing in and promoting new technology has allowed many doctors to administer fast, seemingly definitive tests that tell patients, even asymptomatic ones, whether they may be at risk for a coronary event. The tests have great appeal to patient-consumers interested in thwarting a potential health problem because they are not only noninvasive, but also fast. At least one study has shown the latest version of the CT scan (the 64-slice scanners, which capture an uninterrupted image of the beating heart) to be accurate in giving definitive results faster than conventional stress testing among low-risk patients complaining of chest pains (Raff & Goldstein, 2007). Because of the noninvasive nature of the test and the compelling imagery decipherable to even the layperson, some suggest that tests such as a CT scan of the heart may also give patients better incentives to comply better with physician advice (Berenson & Abelson, 2008). Some physicians may even conclude that the latest

CT scan can save time and money, aid patient education, and even save costs in the long run (Raff & Goldstein, 2007).

Despite this promise, the data on whether these tests can be seen as a value-added step in preventative medicine are hotly contested, and so is their use, especially when ordered in conjunction with older, more traditional tests (Ladapo et al., 2009). Hospitals may worry that patient-consumers will go elsewhere if they cannot offer the latest technology. Hospitals that find themselves in a favorable reimbursement environment might be more likely to invest in the technology (Berwick, 2003; Ladapo et al., 2009; Teplensky, Pauly, Kimberly, Hillman, & Schwartz, 1995).

Concerned that providers are pushing expensive technology that does not truly promote evidence-based medical decisions, insurers and the government have started to adopt guidelines and pay-for-performance schemes based upon physician and technician adherence to a set of established clinical guidelines (Swayne, 2005). Conflict often arises around which guidelines are appropriate, as different constituency groups promote different sets. Historically speaking, associations and institutes representing physicians and specialties such as cardiology have long published guidelines for their members; yet the joint cardiovascular practice guidelines of the ACC and the American Heart Association have come under increasing scrutiny. A recent study revealed that a large number of these guidelines (a little less than one-half) are based on evidence that is considered to be relatively weak (Tricoci, Allen, Kramer, Califf, & Smith, 2009). More pointedly, physicians and academics have criticized guidelines promoted by insurers and other purchasers as being only remotely fashioned after the most recent evidence-based medicine (Steinberg & Luce, 2005).

Societies that represent cardiologists and the technologies in question have vigorously resisted government and private efforts to impose guidelines or limitations on spending for these tests. A group of cardiologists recently sued Secretary of Health and Human Services Kathleen Sebelius over Medicare fee cuts for procedures such as echocardiograms and nuclear stress tests (Sternberg, 2009). Additionally, in response to fee cuts, the American Society of Echocardiography (ASE) ramped up its advocacy efforts to fight private-payer precertification for echocardiography. It is also seeking to preserve Medicare reimbursements for the diagnostic technology. In a statement on the ASE Web site, the Society thanked members for making generous contributions toward this effort (ASE, 2010).

Linking reimbursements to performance as measured by clinical outcomes has had mixed reviews as far as the literature is concerned. An early study on the influence of one pay-for-performance pilot project run by the Centers for Medicare & Medicaid Services (CMS) showed little to no improvement in quality of care for patients with acute myocardial infarction (Glickman et al., 2007). Subsequent studies have shown that pay-for-performance programs—and not only CMS pay-for-performance programs—have influenced notable improvements in other areas of medicine (O'Kane, 2007). Many other studies and literature reviews reveal that evidence on the matter is still scarce or inconclusive (Mehrotra, Damberg, Sorbero, & Teleki, 2009; Petersen, Woodard, Urech, Daw, & Sookanan, 2006; Rosenthal, Frank, Li, & Epstein, 2005). It is not surprising, therefore, that a hospital system and other types of providers may try to avoid certain aspects of the pay-for-performance programs. Negotiating contracts that specifically tie reimbursements to a set of guidelines could be simply putting a provider at a financial disadvantage. Finally, not all physicians unequivocally accept the conclusions of the Dartmouth Data without skepticism. Some would argue that the intensive medicine practiced in high-spending enclaves actually does extend life in chronically ill heart patients with many comorbidities (Langberg & Black, 2009).

Perhaps it is too early to know precisely how different approaches to medicine create or remedy inefficiencies. Despite the burgeoning interest in appropriate-care medicine, the literature and research targeting inequities, inefficiencies, and inappropriate care are not necessarily the drivers behind the appropriateness criteria. Thomas Jones, the health system negotiator from our case vignette, believes that, more often than not, the Dartmouth Data and similar research are misused by insurers to arbitrarily negotiate for lower reimbursements, without evidence of savings or better health outcomes. In more than one conversation that we had with Mr. Jones, he labeled pay-for-performance as "just another scam."

The insurers may refer to the data as part of a drive to reduce reimbursements. And the hospitals that know what they are doing will use it as a way to increase their price. . . . There is an underlying criticism that doctors do too much, or that patients want too much because of defensive medicine. And if you took away defensive medicine everyone would get appropriate care. I'm telling you that we don't know what appropriate care is. . . . I am going to fight every effort that limits care to people who aren't sick, but who maybe [sic] sick. Because there is no one out there who definitively knows who should have that cardiogram, or that MRI, that surgery or that chemotherapy.

At this point in the exercise I ask a few volunteers to do a quick role-play simulation. I assign different groups to represent different stakeholders in a fictitious case vignette. Some represent hospital negotiators, others play a group of "in-house" cardiologists associated with a large network of hospitals, and some are tasked with representing the insurers. If the size of the group warrants it, I might also assign some volunteers to represent physicians working independently, the news media, government bodies, and patient advocacy groups. With a smaller group, however, I ask them to consider the value proposition of the following five influences, but rather than simply assigning them a certain value I ask them to prioritize the influences in order of importance. Sometimes I present the exercise like this:

As far as value creation is concerned, all of these influences are important. But as a stakeholder you have limited resources and time and must decide how to prioritize these items given that you are in the middle of a time-sensitive negotiation. These are the issues at hand: (a) better health outcomes, (b) how news media portrays your actions, (c) increasing coverage for treatment (which is also thought of as access), (d) patient, or "customer," satisfaction, (e) adequate revenue for services rendered.

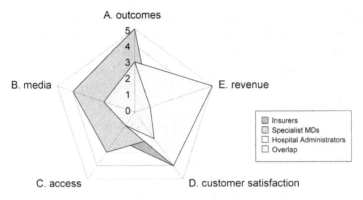

FIGURE 6.2 Mapping out alignment.

Then I ask the participants to rank these in order of importance, with "5" being the strongest and "1" being the least important. No item can be given the same importance as any other in this exercise.

Figure 6.2 shows the result when I ran this simulation with a few of my colleagues playing the roles of different stakeholders. I would point out that this is an exercise of role-play, not the mapping of a real-life scenario. The first observation from the result is that there is very little overlap. Also, the overlap may be skewed, reflecting the various priorities of the different stakeholders. Overlap is represented by the shape at the center of the diagram. By using spider plots we have come across a unique visual effect. It is compelling because this mapping exercise lets each stakeholder see just how far away he or she is from alignment with other stakeholders and their priorities. Often, I find that a stakeholder may hold on too tightly to a particular agenda that he or she may feel must be prioritized above all other issues; or perhaps a stakeholder may not be able to "see" clearly the priorities of another stakeholder, making negotiations difficult due to a certain level of misunderstanding.

Past literature on stakeholder theory helps managers think strategically about how powerful and influential other stakeholders are in different scenarios. Saliency modeling also helped them become aware of those who may be smaller and therefore less obvious, but nonetheless influential, entities (Savage, Nix, Whitehead, & Blair, 1991). One book published in 1990 guided readers to create lists of various stakeholders. In different instances, the authors showed how stakeholder groups were varied and diverse, and the book offered comparisons of one type of hospital ecology to another (Blair & Fottler, 1990).

Other work on stakeholder alignment, such as that mentioned in Chapter 5, has concentrated more on saliency. Stakeholder saliency in business parlance has come to mean evaluating three elements: power, legitimacy, and criticality (Mitchell, Agle, & Wood, 1997). In many ways, stakeholder theory has stressed the importance of identifying the key stakeholders and thinking strategically about handling these stakeholders and their possible influences. Here, I want to revive the basic spirit in which stakeholder theory was first conceived by Edward Freeman and colleagues, one that assigned a normative and prescriptive aspect to stakeholder behavior.

Freeman et al. (2007) spoke of a "philosophy of voluntarism" in which stakeholders self-manage, without the hand of government or other large entities overseeing them. They also called for an "intensive dialogue" between stakeholders, and for the generalizing of the "marketing approach." Among other things, they said that "a constant monitoring of processes" was needed to better serve all the stakeholders (Freeman, Harrison, & Wicks, 2007). Value is inherently knotted into the stakeholders and the stakeholder relationships, but accessing that value is challenging because many stakeholders cannot see past their conflicting priorities. Furthermore, smaller stakeholders may be at the periphery of the Gordian knot, but that does not mean they would not be able to derail the value-creation process.

We like to refer to a definition of "a stakeholder" put forward by Grossi (2003), a student of lean enterprise thinking and stakeholder theory whom we mentioned earlier in this chapter. His work centered on analyzing stakeholders from a "systems dynamics approach." This is an approach that incorporates a global analysis of a particular ecosystem. In the business and science worlds, it has often been applied to analyze how various elements and entities may influence one another. In his Master's thesis, Grossi (2003) looked at how to define stakeholders and the concept of value within a business environment that takes into account all the potential contributors, large and small. His definition is below:

[A] stakeholder is any group or individual who directly or indirectly affects or is affected by the level of achievement of an enterprise's value creation process.

In this book, we relate the notion of stakeholder value and the value-creation process back to the health care environment. Here is our definition of value from a stakeholder perspective:

A stakeholder is a group or an individual who directly or indirectly influences health outcomes in striving to create value for the patient.

We want to be clear that the patient is not excluded from this definition. Indeed, the patient can be a very active stakeholder who may choose to derail the whole value-creation process, or augment it, by pursuing or shunning a healthier lifestyle or adhering to sound advice from health care providers. In the next section, we focus on the nature of value creation between health care stakeholders and how it can be augmented by Lean principles. If appropriated deliberately, Lean principles can help health care stakeholders align, or simply see the possibility for aligning their priorities.

6.4 STAKEHOLDER THEORY IN THE CONTEXT OF LEAN ENTERPRISE THINKING

Negotiations between stakeholders (and the decisions that eventuate from the discussions) have the potential to either augment or erode value. Having clearly defined guiding principles can be useful in deciding whether certain decisions, attitudes, priorities, and approaches can have a positive or negative impact on creating value. When considering Lean enterprise, one has to be cautious, because often the audience may have very strong, preconceived ideas about what constitutes "Lean." Many people may associate "Lean processes" with uncomfortable change, cutbacks in staff, and expensive consultants. For example, numerous hospitals across the United States have hired consultants to expedite the processing of patient admission to busy emergency departments. Some of these efforts have incorporated Lean analysis and proven successful. Some, however, have not been successful, depending on how the process changes were instituted and whether the stakeholders involved were actively brought into the efforts. Here, we are not going to discuss specifics of process improvement influenced by Lean thinking, which involves careful calculations and the continual study of the situation. Instead, we are taking a hard look at the philosophy behind Lean thinking when it comes to seeking stakeholder alignment, especially in the health care environment.

Classic Lean thinking incorporates ideas that are perhaps best summarized by James P. Womack and Daniel T. Jones, who co-wrote a series of books explaining the seemingly miraculous success of the Toyota Production System pioneered by Taiichi Ohno (Ohno, 1988; Womack & Jones, 1996; Womack, Jones, & Roos, 1990). To summarize (and to simplify slightly), they proposed that an enterprise engaging in Lean thinking was to first establish and specify "value" from the customer's perspective. Secondly, enterprises and stakeholders are to identify and map out the steps that exist in the creation of value. Thirdly, these steps need to come in fast sequential order, and wasteful steps that do not add value need to be eliminated. Fourthly, customers need to be able to "pull" value from the producer. Finally, the process is perfected and repeated, with careful attention paid to wasteful steps and the pulling of value.

A simple circular diagram, which we interpret and reproduce in Figure 6.3, summarizes this breakdown, but this depiction can also be accessed in its original form on a Web site created by author James P. Womack to promote his Lean Enterprise Institute (The Lean Enterprise Institute, 2009). We want to emphasize that what we might distill from this diagram is where and how stakeholders can seek alignment with these Lean principles. In Chapter 1, we quoted Professor Earll Murman and his co-authors, who mentioned how adding value is only possible when there is mutual agreement, which may be either tacit or implicit (Murman et al., 2002a).

Getting started on true value creation in the world of health care is difficult. This is where a few tried-and-true Lean thinking tools can help. Borrowing from the five Lean principles diagrammed in Figure 6.3, we are posing the following six questions to health care stakeholders in any given scenario or situation:

1. Can the health care stakeholders establish and specify "value" in terms of outcomes or a better quality of living for patients?
2. Are the stakeholders able to identify and map out an agreed-upon route with specific steps toward the previously agreed-upon value?

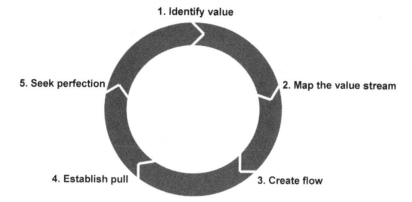

FIGURE 6.3 Classic Lean Enterprise thinking. Adapted from "What is Lean" by J.P. Womack, 2009, The Lean Enterprise Institute. Principles of Lean. Retrieved August 26, 2010 from http://www.lean.org/WhatsLean/Principles.cfm.

3. Are there barriers to these steps for one or more particular stakeholders (e.g., high costs, market-related barriers, legal and privacy barriers, etc.) that might prohibit a clear direction (e.g., the flow)?
4. Can the stakeholders agree upon what steps may be wasteful and therefore need to be eliminated?
5. Can each stakeholder group help patients better manage their health in the short and long term through better education and the coordination of care delivery?
6. Are there reliable benchmarks that can be used to gauge health improvement in terms of patient well-being, morbidity and mortality outcomes, cost savings, participation, and feedback from the patient's side? (This last question encompasses the Lean principle of "pull," which seeks to let the customer [in this case the patient] add value to care.)

If we take a moment to think back to our case vignette, we can see how the stakeholders obviously had different motivations; yet their priorities were not too far from being closely aligned. In our role-play exercise, alignment seemed a distant possibility. This is something that we established by mapping out the fictitious stakeholders' priorities. However, if we look back at the real stakeholders in the case vignette, they were constantly pursuing continued communication and were dedicated to finding common ground despite the strong differences in their approaches to creating value. If we consider that value for the patient can be found in improved health outcomes, and perhaps also in a better quality of life through decreased morbidity or improved chronic disease management, then all the stakeholders in our exercise may align themselves easily.

When we engage in a scenario of stakeholder role-play, it becomes clear that there are many paths up the same mountain; I have run this role-play exercise where all the volunteers prioritized health outcomes, for example. An interesting discussion ensued, with observers in the classroom saying that while everyone desires improved health outcomes, they saw no immediately actionable items in such a time-sensitive scenario that would really impact outcomes. Another observer commented that outcomes are particular to the population of a hospital or the community it serves, and therefore data on outcomes may be inconsistent or easily influenced by outside factors that providers may not be able to control. With that particular group of role-playing volunteers, I would say that there seemed to be great potential for creating long-term alignment in creating better value for patients. But I have also encountered a group where all the volunteers wanted to preserve customer satisfaction as the utmost priority because they were mainly motivated by the fear of losing market share.

As we mentioned earlier, customer satisfaction does not necessarily move in tandem with better patient outcomes. In such a situation, more long-term thinking needs to be applied, and a deeper analysis of customer satisfaction needs to be undertaken. Does this mean higher satisfaction among an increasingly dwindling group of individuals with excellent insurance coverage? We know from our literature review in the earlier chapters that an intensive, invasive, and even defensive type of medicine may satiate the demanding customer-patient—but this does not bring better health outcomes to the wider population, and it increases costs for all patients and all other stakeholders. Generally speaking, purchasers and the health insurance companies have not been effective at reigning in rising health costs while also ensuring improving outcomes (although there are some exceptions to this generalization, which we will discuss in the next chapter).

For a moment, we want to zero in on one key element of Lean enterprise thinking, and that is what is meant by the "value proposition" between stakeholders, summarized by Professor Murman and colleagues (2002b). With this proposition comes a question that begs an honest and aligned view of "value" among the stakeholders: does every stakeholder have the "sufficient capability" to succeed at every agreed-upon task at hand? Understanding a stakeholder's "capacity" is a major step in arriving at the value proposition (Murman et al., 2002b). Oftentimes, mistrust between stakeholders comes not only from negative experiences of past interactions, but also from assumptions about fellow stakeholders' present and future ability and capacity to fulfill a particular promise. Because doubts enter the fray about long-term planning and ability to commit to long-term planning, stakeholders are likely to focus on the short-term ideas on cost-cutting measures and boosting satisfaction.

Let us relate this back, once again, to the "Tragedy of the Commons" put forward by Garrett Hardin (1968). In the game-theory scenario suggested by Hardin, herdsmen share a common pasture. We would find that the difficulty of managing this common resource arises not because the herdsmen do not recognize the value in sharing the pasture; quite the contrary—they recognize that sharing the pasture promotes sustained growth. The difficulty arises because there is a temptation to "cheat," and with this there is also mistrust. This mistrust arises because there is a chance that cheaters will initially be rewarded by higher profits if they add more cattle and then exit the game by selling their entire herd, thus escaping the consequences as the pasture collapses from overuse.

We want to emphasize that trust is an element in the sustained management of a common resource, but arriving at a point where trust is possible is the main challenge faced by stakeholders in health care (Shore, 2005, 2007). We are not asking stakeholders to blindly trust in one another. A major tenet of Lean thinking is continued and sustained interaction, communication, and verification (Murman et al., 2002b). This goes beyond simply building trust with other stakeholders—we are advocating that stakeholders do their homework. They must stay aware of the trends and developing values of their fellow stakeholders (Murman et al., 2002b; Shore, 2007). This requires a learned competency of fostering deep and sustained information exchange between stakeholders—even among stakeholders who have seen themselves as competitors in the past.

In the next chapter, we present another case vignette, in which a large purchaser is working very closely with other stakeholders not only to establish a great deal of trust, but also to control health care costs through the fostering of preventative medicine and a healthier lifestyle among its beneficiaries. Toward the end of the next chapter, we evaluate the value proposition among the stakeholders involved.

REFERENCES

Abelson, R. (2006, August 18). Heart procedure is off the charts in an Ohio city. *New York Times*, p. A1.

American Society of Echocardiography. (2010). *Breaking News Archives*. Retrieved 2010, from http://www.asecho.org/i4a/headlines/headlinearchives.cfm

Berenson, A., & Abelson, R. (2008, June 29). Weighing the costs of a CT scan's look inside the heart. *New York Times*, p. A1.

Berwick, D. M. (2003). Disseminating innovations in health care. *Journal of the American Medical Association, 289*(15), 1969–1975.

Blair, J. D., & Fottler, M. D. (1990). *Challenges in health care management: Strategic perspectives for managing key stakeholders* (1st ed.). San Francisco, CA: Jossey-Bass.

Block, M. (Writer). (2009). Doctors say costs, not care, have become focus [radio broadcast]. *Health care overhaul: Prescriptions for change*. USA: National Public Radio.

Brenner, D. J., & Hall, E. J. (2007). Computed tomography—an increasing source of radiation exposure. *New England Journal of Medicine, 357*(22), 2277–2284.

Brownlee, S. (2003, March 16). The perils of prevention. *New York Times*.

The Dartmouth Institute for Health Policy & Clinical Practice. (2009). The Dartmouth Atlas of Health Care. Retrieved December 2, 2010, from http://www.dartmouthatlas.org/

DeSantis, A. (2008, June 29). The unnecessary expense: A case study. *New York Times*. Available at http://www.nytimes.com/imagepages/2008/06/29/business/29scan.graph1.web.html

Fisher, E., Goodman, D., Skinner, J., & Bronner, K. (2009). *Health care spending, quality, and outcomes: More isn't always better*. Hanover, NH: Dartmouth Institute for Health Policy and Clinical Practice.

Fisher, E. S. (2003). Medical care—is more always better? *New England Journal of Medicine, 349*(17), 1665–1667.

Fisher, E. S., Wennberg, D. E., Stukel, T. A., Gottlieb, D. J., Lucas, F. L., & Pinder, E. L. (2003a). The implications of regional variations in Medicare spending. Part 1: The content, quality, and accessibility of care. *Annals of Internal Medicine, 138*(4), 273–287.

Fisher, E. S., Wennberg, D. E., Stukel, T. A., Gottlieb, D. J., Lucas, F. L., & Pinder, E. L. (2003b). The implications of regional variations in Medicare spending. Part 2: Health outcomes and satisfaction with care. *Annals of Internal Medicine, 138*(4), 288–298.

Freeman, R. E., Harrison, J. S., & Wicks, A. C. (2007). *Managing for stakeholders: Survival, reputation and success* (pp. 47–73). New Haven, CT: Yale University Press.

Gawande, A., Berwick, D., Fisher, E., & McClellan, M. (2009, August 12). 10 steps to better health care. *New York Times*, p. A27.

Glabman, M. (2005). Health plans strain to contain rapidly rising cost of imaging. *Managed Care, 14*(1), 22–24, 26, 28; passim.

Glickman, S. W., Ou, F. S., DeLong, E. R., Roe, M. T., Lytle, B. L., Mulgund, J., et al. (2007). Pay for performance, quality of care, and outcomes in acute myocardial infarction. *Journal of the American Medical Association, 297*(21), 2373–2380.

Grossi, I. (2003). *Stakeholder analysis in the context of the lean enterprise*. Unpublished master's thesis, Massachusetts Institute of Technology, Cambridge.

Hardin, G. (1968). The tragedy of the commons. *Science, 162*(5364), 1243–1248.

Hendel, R. C. (2008). The revolution and evolution of appropriateness in cardiac imaging. *Journal of Nuclear Cardiology, 15*(4), 494–496.

Heron, M., Hoyert, D. L., Murphy, S. L., Xu, J., Kochanek, K. D., & Tejada-Vera, B. (2009). Deaths: Final data for 2006. *National Vital Statistics Reports, 57*(14), 1–134.

Ladapo, J. A., Horwitz, J. R., Weinstein, M. C., Gazelle, G. S., & Cutler, D. M. (2009). Adoption and spread of new imaging technology: A case study. *Health Affairs (Millwood), 28*(6), w1122–w1132.

Langberg, M. L., & Black, J. T. (2009). Dead souls—comparing Dartmouth Atlas benchmarks with CMS outcomes data. *New England Journal of Medicine, 361*(22), e109.

The Lean Enterprise Institute. Principles of Lean. Retrieved November 24, 2009, from http://www.lean.org/whatslean/principles.cfm

Mahoney, J., & Hom, D. (2006). *Total value total return: Seven rules for optimizing employee health benefits for a healthier and more productive workforce*. Philadelphia: GlaxoSmithKline.

Mehrotra, A., Damberg, C. L., Sorbero, M. E., & Teleki, S. S. (2009). Pay for performance in the hospital setting: What is the state of the evidence? *American Journal of Medical Quality, 24*(1), 19–28.

Mitchell, R. K., Agle, B. R., & Wood, D. J. (1997). Toward a theory of stakeholder identification and salience: Defining the principle of who and what really counts. *Academy of Management Review, 22*(4), 853–886.

Murman, E., Allen, T., Bozdogan, K., Cutcher-Gershenfeld, J., McManus, H., Nightingale, D., et al. (2002a). The 21st century enterprise challenge. In *Lean enterprise value: Insights from MIT's aerospace initiative* (p. 9). New York: Palgrave.

Murman, E., Allen, T., Bozdogan, K., Cutcher-Gershenfeld, J., McManus, H., Nightingale, D., et al. (2002b). Value at national and international levels. In *Lean enterprise value: Insights from MIT's lean aerospace initiative* (pp. 247–280). New York: Palgrave.

O'Kane, M. E. (2007). Performance-based measures: The early results are in. *Journal of Managed Care Pharmacy, 13*(2 Suppl B), S3–S6.

Ohno, T. (1988). *Toyota production system: Beyond large-scale production*. New York: Productivity Press.

Petersen, L. A., Woodard, L. D., Urech, T., Daw, C., & Sookanan, S. (2006). Does pay-for-performance improve the quality of health care? *Annals of Internal Medicine, 145*(4), 265–272.

Porter, M. E., & Teisberg, E. O. (2006). Strategic implications for health care providers. In *Redefining healthcare: Creating value based competition on results* (pp. 149–228). Boston: Harvard Business School Press.

Raff, G. L., & Goldstein, J. A. (2007). Coronary angiography by computed tomography: Coronary imaging evolves. *Journal of the American College of Cardiology, 49*(18), 1830–1833.

Rosenthal, M. B., Frank, R. G., Li, Z., & Epstein, A. M. (2005). Early experience with pay-for-performance: From concept to practice. *Journal of the American Medical Association, 294*(14), 1788–1793.

Savage, G. T., Nix, T. W., Whitehead, C. J., & Blair, J. D. (1991). Strategies for assessing and managing organizational stakeholders. *The Executive, 5*(2), 61–75.

Seidel, R. L., & Nash, D. B. (2004). Paying for performance in diagnostic imaging: Current challenges and future prospects. *Journal of the American College of Radiology, 1*(12), 952–956.

Shore, D. A. (2005). *The trust prescription for healthcare: Building your reputation with consumers*. Chicago: Health Administration Press.

Shore, D. A. (Ed.). (2007). *The trust crisis in healthcare: Causes, consequences, and cures* (1st ed.). New York: Oxford University Press.

Smith-Bindman, R., Miglioretti, D. L., & Larson, E. B. (2008). Rising use of diagnostic medical imaging in a large integrated health system. *Health Affairs (Millwood), 27*(6), 1491–1502.

Solomon, M. D., Goldman, D. P., Joyce, G. F., & Escarce, J. J. (2009). Cost sharing and the initiation of drug therapy for the chronically ill. *Archives of Internal Medicine, 169*(8), 740–748; discussion 748–749.

Steinberg, E. P., & Luce, B. R. (2005). Evidence based? Caveat emptor! *Health Affairs (Millwood), 24*(1), 80–92.

Sternberg, S. (2009, December 28). Cardiologists sue Sebelius over Medicare fee cuts. *USA Today*.

Studdert, D. M., Mello, M. M., Sage, W. M., DesRoches, C. M., Peugh, J., Zapert, K., et al. (2005). Defensive medicine among high-risk specialist physicians in a volatile malpractice environment. *Journal of the American Medical Association, 293*(21), 2609–2617.

Swayne, L. C. (2005). Pay for performance: Pay more or pay less? *Journal of the American College of Radiology, 2*(9), 777–781.

Teplensky, J. D., Pauly, M. V., Kimberly, J. R., Hillman, A. L., & Schwartz, J. S. (1995). Hospital adoption of medical technology: An empirical test of alternative models. *Health Services Research, 30*(3), 437–465.

Tricoci, P., Allen, J. M., Kramer, J. M., Califf, R. M., & Smith, S. C., Jr. (2009). Scientific evidence underlying the ACC/AHA clinical practice guidelines. *Journal of the American Medical Association, 301*(8), 831–841.

U.S. Government Accountability Office. (2008). *Medicare part B imaging services: Rapid spending growth and shift to physician offices indicate need for CMS to consider additional management practices* (No. GAO-08-452). Washington, DC: U.S. Government Accountability Office.

Van Decker, W. (2009, May 15). *Regarding the Senate Finance Committee's Health Reform Policy Options: Transforming the Health Care Delivery System: Proposals to Improve Patient Care and Reduce Health Care Costs* [Open Letter]. Retrieved June 19, 2009, from American Society of Nuclear Cardiology website: http://www.asnc.org/

Wennberg, D. E., & Wennberg, J. E. (2003). Addressing variations: Is there hope for the future? *Health Affairs (Millwood),* Web Exclusives, W3-614–617.

Wennberg, J. E., Bronner, K., Skinner, J. S., Fisher, E. S., & Goodman, D. C. (2009). Inpatient care intensity and patients' ratings of their hospital experiences. *Health Affairs (Millwood), 28*(1), 103–112.

Womack, J. P., & Jones, D. T. (1996). *Lean thinking: Banish waste and create wealth in your corporation.* New York: Free Press.

Womack, J. P., Jones, D. T., & Roos, D. (1990). *The machine that changed the world: The story of lean production.* New York: Rawson Associates.

Yasaitis, L., Fisher, E., Mackenzie, T. A., & Wasson, J. (2009). Healthcare intensity is associated with lower ratings of healthcare quality by younger adults. *Journal of Ambulatory Care Management, 32*(3), 226–231.

7 Working toward Better Health and Greater Satisfaction

7.1 SEARCHING FOR COST SAVINGS

In contrast to most other places in the world, the employers, as a whole, are a major purchaser of health care services in the United States. Virtually all of these employers have looked for relief from rising health care costs with increasing desperation in recent years. Some have turned to outside consultants for assistance. Still others have invested time and money to bring in their own staff to develop cost-controlling measures. For these concerned employers, traditional strategies include shifting an increasing proportion of the health benefit cost burden to employees in the form of higher co-payments, higher deductibles, and/or curtailing some portion of coverage such as pharmaceutical benefits. Their newer strategies include moving to coinsurance, mandating the use of generics, or placing utilization-management restrictions (such as step therapy and prior authorization) on pharmacy benefits.

Many other employers have sought greater bargaining power by joining local, regional, and/or national (business) coalitions in order to secure lower prices on a range of health services from both providers and suppliers. Still others have invested in efforts to create a culture of healthier living among their employees in the hopes of saving money by lowering employee morbidities. Such efforts may include, for example, a wellness program, a discounted or "free" pass to health clubs, and extended access to an on-site doctor. Then there is the even smaller number of companies that have implemented the above *and* rethought healthcare purchasing altogether. They have made longer-term commitments toward securing better health outcomes over the working lifetime of their employee population. In the course of putting together this next case vignette, I spoke to a great number of professionals from different stakeholder groups of various sizes, from the quite small to the very large.

One of the first individuals I spoke to when researching this book is heavily involved in securing lower costs for larger companies that participate in purchasing coalitions. Interesting, though, is his background: Larry Boress worked for the Illinois State Medical Society for seventeen years before transferring his skills to a completely different area of health care. His former work largely entailed lobbying for the interests of the state's local doctors. His career changed directions entirely in the early 1990s when he found "something on the opposite side of the fence." He decided that instead of working for the providers, he would take a position representing the purchaser community. Mr. Boress began his new career with a nonprofit business coalition called Midwest Business Group on Health (MBGH), in 1991, and has since gone on to become the group's president and CEO. I first met Larry Boress when he attended a stakeholder workshop I led in Chicago.

The nonprofit packs a sizable punch. It started out with members that were typically large Midwest manufacturers, such as Honeywell, General Mills, and Motorola. Today, MBGH's corporate members number more than 100. These firms provide benefits to about two million people, and in dollar terms the employee populations together represent health care spending in the range of $2 billion per year. In addition to its national efforts, MBGH also helps its members form local coalitions Detroit, Milwaukee, Columbus, and other cities throughout the Midwest. For the most part, MBGH does not represent smaller or medium-sized firms with fewer beneficiaries. On average, a member might have about three thousand employees, which translates to about eight to nine thousand health care beneficiaries.

While MBGH holds activities such as conferences and educational forums, one major benefit that members receive comes from its benchmarking efforts. MBGH gives its members a bird's-eye view of provider trends in reimbursements. For large employers, this could mean better bargaining power, which may translate into cost savings. Some members are looking also to form "purchasing groups" in order to influence reimbursement negotiations by augmenting collective bargaining power. Additionally, MBGH operates a research arm that looks at a vast array of topics, among them activities that influence beneficiaries' behavior in health-related decisions. Some of these activities also come in the form of incentives, punitive and otherwise, geared toward enticing beneficiaries to make healthier choices. This carrot-and-stick approach aims to encourage healthier lifestyles, better disease self-management, and, therefore, lower morbidity rates.

A wave of literature has surfaced in recent years on how purchasers may bring about better health outcomes for their employee populations using the "carrot" approach of incentives. The main driver behind this thinking is that healthier, more productive employees can ultimately lead to employer savings in both the short and long term. Pitney Bowes, whose activities have influenced numerous other business and educational endeavors, published its own version of how stakeholders may bring value to health care beneficiaries and, in turn, savings to health care purchasers. They advocate some general strategies, summarized in seven steps for encouraging healthier employee lifestyles and better disease management. The strategies are presented for purchasers in an easy-to-adopt format that emphasizes human capital (employee base) as an important company resource (Mahoney & Hom, 2006).

These and other efforts at understanding worksite wellness have influenced a number of medium- and large-sized corporations in recent years who are looking to reduce the direct and indirect costs of illness. Direct costs may be associated with serious, progressive illnesses such as cancer and cardiovascular disease—the health problems that typically account for highest proportion of a firm's health care spending (Hemp, 2004). But an increasing number of firms have started to examine chronic and episodic health problems that may cost little to treat when compared to the large and unknown or hidden costs suffered in terms of worker productivity (Burton, Chen, Conti, Schultz, & Edington, 2003; Burton, Morrison, & Wertheimer, 2003; Goetzel et al., 2004). This broader notion has been best captured in the use of the word "presenteeism"—employees not only miss work but also are less productive when they are present on the job (Hilton, Scuffham, Sheridan, Cleary, & Whiteford, 2008; Kessler et al., 2004; Wang et al., 2003). For employers attuned to this concern, the lost productivity represents a cost that is hidden but very real. Several tools have emerged that try to capture productivity losses due to on-the-job employee morbidity.

My colleague Professor Ronald Kessler, at Harvard Medical School, proposed one such method to look at overall worker performance. The tool has received one of the highest levels of endorsement, having been adopted by the World Health Organization and numerous businesses (Hemp, 2004; Kessler et al., 2004). Professor Kessler and his colleagues have continued to show that worker health and productivity are related and carry serious implications for employers (Loeppke et al., 2009; Loeppke et al., 2007). While Professor Kessler's research has burgeoned into a field of its own, other entities, such as the Institute for Health and Productivity Management, have endeavored to create robust tools for corporations looking to quantify and curb productivity loss due to illness.

7.2 THE NEXT WAVE OF HEALTH CARE PURCHASER COST MANAGEMENT

The next case vignette is about a company that has made a very extensive investment in increasing health care access and improving interventional strategies against illness for its workforce. This company has drawn on myriad ideas, tools, and philosophies and has contracted with several partners to implement this approach. When I spoke to key figures from both the firm and participating stakeholders, the program was still in its infancy. As we go to press, the possible cost-savings benefits from healthier lifestyles and lower morbidity have not yet been fully realized. That is what makes this example compelling, especially regarding the expectations of all the stakeholders involved. We have an opportunity to witness whether a well-planned endeavor targeting employee health will bring the benefits that are hoped for.

We mentioned previously that a great many companies have introduced wellness programs for their employees. These companies have enlisted on-site physicians, created clinics, and brought in mobile screening units for regular health checks. Other organizations have offered free or subsidized health and fitness classes. But some companies have done this and much more: they have approached investing in employee health as a critical element in an overall strategy for holding down labor costs. We spoke to several executives at Towers Watson (formerly Towers Perrin), a global professional services company focused on improving staff effectiveness, risk mitigation, and financial management. For our purposes, we will focus on Towers Watson's initiatives to help companies better control health care costs.

I spoke to one enthusiastic executive, Dave Guilmette, who for many years was managing director for Towers Watson's health and group benefits practice, until he left the firm early in 2010 to become President, National Segment president at CIGNA. In conversations with Mr. Guilmette, we learned his views about which firms are likely to have the resources to make long-term employee-centered health-related commitments. He explained that mid-sized to large employers are best positioned for such investments. He suggested that smaller firms have a disadvantage because they may not be able to make the large capital outlays deemed necessary to implement system-wide changes:

Customized solutions to managing employee health and productivity often require significant resources, including capital outlay. Those with fewer than 1000 employees are significantly challenged to make the economics work. These smaller companies are confined to working with product solutions that are more off the shelf. And while those are effective to a point, they don't fully optimize program performance for the characteristics of a company's specific employee population, profile or culture which is essentially to ultimately curb rising costs.

For companies that can afford a larger investment, there are great cost savings to be had, according to Mr. Guilmette. He explained that among other activities, Towers Watson conducts a comprehensive annual health care cost survey. Previously, this survey grouped survey participants into two categories: "high performing" and "low performing." Among the attributes used to define whether or not a company is high performing is a company's per capita cost for delivering the medical benefits. Mr. Guilmette reported that the data gathered are adjusted for design, demographic, and geographic differences among corporate beneficiary plans.

Typically, highperforming companies seem to have invested in the expertise to look strategically at curbing morbidity as a means of holding down costs, explained Mr. Guilmette: "You are seeing results that are really quite different, there is about a $1,500 per capita cost-difference, for example, between the high performing and the low performing companies." Companies that are large, and those that typically appear in the Fortune 500, or even Fortune 1000, lists are more likely also to be seen as "high performing." He noted that for such companies the prospect of continuing to play a large role in health care purchasing is really part of their long-term competitive strategy. These organizations remain committed to playing an active role in managing wellness and employee health for their workforce going forward:

> High performing organizations are producing far better results and gaining a competitive advantage over those that are not. These companies would not want to get out of their role in managing wellness and employee health as long as they are doing a good job, and producing competitive advantage when doing so.

One of the many companies Towers Watson has worked with is Cisco Systems, Inc. This company started its own comprehensive system of care in 2006, with planned annual expansions. It was built on the premise that employees (and their families) need to actively engage in certain activities to take care of their health. The program started with a personal health assessment, which integrates Professor Kessler's tools to measure presenteeism with other means of measuring health and risk factors. One area looks directly at the workforce for health risks that could lead to illness and chronic conditions. Cisco offered about $300 to entice employees to participate in the health assessment; this was in preparation for a much bigger and flashier investment.

In 2008, Cisco opened a sizable on-site health care facility on its main campus, in San Jose, California. The facility targets Cisco's employees and their dependents. Strategically, its main function is to provide a "medical home" where many different aspects of health care are integrated into practice. The concept of the "medical home" may be found as early as the 1960s in a book published by the American Academy of Pediatrics (Sia, Tonniges, Osterhus, & Taba, 2004). Back then, the Academy envisioned a sort of progressive primary care facility for infants and children. Such a facility would maintain a complete and centralized medical record for each individual. In recent years, the concept of a medical home has developed to mean a place of primary and coordinated care, with an emphasis on the integrated management of health for individuals and families (Sia et al., 2004).

Different stakeholders may have varying definitions about what constitutes a medical home. For Cisco Systems, the definition includes many different aspects. For example, quite apart from providing on-site primary care, Cisco has looked to tailor the care to the employee population. A large proportion of their engineers and staff are of South Asian origin and expressed a desire for therapies that originated in Asia, such as acupuncture. Physical therapy, chiropractic care, and nutritionists have also been made available at the health site.

The lead architect and overseer of this program is Dr. Pamela Hymel. In her role as senior director of Integrated Health and corporate medical director for Cisco Systems, she looks after the present and future health needs of approximately sixty thousand employees worldwide. In addition to the approximately seventeen thousand employees on the firm's main campus in the San Jose, California, area, there are nearly forty-five thousand employees and dependents who rely on Cisco's benefits package in San Jose alone. Dr. Hymel is a champion of preventive medicine and a strong believer that she can impact Cisco's workforce in such a way as to actually avoid a great deal of chronic disease. She looks to accomplish this by considering common risk factors and intervening before the small health issues cause bigger health problems that require more invasive and expensive medical attention.

Our average age at Cisco is around 40, and our turnover is very low.... So we know these employees are going to be with us for the long haul and as they age into their 40s and 50s, we thought that this would give us a great opportunity if we began to focus on health risks to see whether we could actually impact the health outcomes of this population. So when we first started our health enhancement program we found that 30% of our employees had two or more health risks for a fairly young population, and that was a concern.

Another reason Cisco built its state-of-the-art on-campus health facility is its strong belief that costs could be better controlled in many areas of care delivery. For example, in promoting better health management, Cisco hopes to cut down on expensive emergency room visits and treatments. By encouraging the use of the on-campus facility, they might possibly redirect users from inappropriate care that is costly yet does not necessarily lead to better outcomes. Cisco also wanted to apply its own technology in managing a "paperless" environment and promoting a seamless approach to health care delivery. In Dr. Hymel's words, the company saw the program as an opportunity not only to improve the long-term health prospects of their workforce, but also to showcase the possible technology-facilitated improvements to health care delivery.

Because of our strong feeling that technology can change the way health care is delivered we wanted to design a clinic that had a paperless environment with automatic check-ins, and immediate feeds to claims administrators for payment.

Cisco pooled data from the past couple of years and loaded them into an integrated database (with the help of a third-party company) to better assess medical-trend costs. Dr. Hymel explained that part of the program's uniqueness is an ability to analyze claims data and "marry" them to data the company collected on productivity through the presenteeism tools mentioned earlier. Dr. Hymel first noticed that a high proportion of beneficiaries live with heart disease, high cholesterol, and hypertension—known risk factors for more serious health problems. There were also data indicating a high rate of musculoskeletal issues. The claims data showed that Cisco's top three costs were pregnancy, musculoskeletal problems, and cancer. However, when Dr. Hymel looked at the health risks and began to merge the information with data gathered on presenteeism, a slightly different picture emerged. Musculoskeletal issues were still a big cost driver, but Dr. Hymel also began to see that problems such as stress, anxiety, and sleeplessness were actually the company's highest cost drivers as far as costs to worker productivity were concerned. In reaction, Dr. Hymel and her team put together a "high touch intervention program" that adopted more Health and Work Performance Questionnaire (HPQ) tools, with one specifically tailored by Professor Kessler (Harvard School of Medicine and United Behavioral Health) to look at employees who self-identify with depression and anxiety (Harvard School of Medicine, 2010). Those who self-identified with such issues were offered help in the form of referrals to counsellors trained to address not only behavioral health issues but also any underlying medical issues that might be contributing to a patient's depression.

While the beneficiaries might find the approach to be one that improves their outlook for leading a happier, healthier, and more productive life, Cisco has also calculated almost immediate cost savings. In the early months of the program, Dr. Hymel and her team made a back-of-the-envelope calculation on savings from improved productivity and lessened absenteeism. By benchmarking savings from figures collected in the first and second years of the program, Cisco estimated a cost savings of nearly $2 million (see Figure 7.1). Dr. Hymel expects the savings to be more noticeable as more beneficiaries take advantage of the programs and facilities offered at the San Jose campus. In many ways, Dr. Hymel hopes to set a new standard for other purchasers looking to improve outcomes through better beneficiary self-management, with Cisco serving as an international leader in this effort.

When Cisco started the program, Dr. Hymel expected significant resistance. She imagined employees saying things like "I don't want to go to a company doctor" or "I don't want Cisco to know about my medical information." To assuage any concerns that may have existed before the program started, Cisco contracted several third-party vendors. For example, Cerner Corporation handles in support of Cisco's electronic medical records and provides administrative staff. Cisco also partnered with a third-party medical group called North First Street Medical Group, which hires and manages the medical care staff, such as the physicians and chiropractors. Dr. Hymel explained that part of the motivation to outsource aspects of this program is to make certain that a highly visible firewall exists between employees' personal medical records and Cisco itself.

Despite these efforts, many users did not immediately avail themselves of the new health facilities and related programs. Dr. Hymel now expects that it might take a while for potential users to switch from their current provider to a new physician on campus. She had hoped the facility itself would wow the employees. For example, the clinic is equipped with some of the latest technology, which allows it to offer a "paperless" visit and expedite the administrative and waiting times typically associated with a trip to the doctor's office. When patients arrive at the Cisco facility, they are quickly signed in and then escorted to one of the fifteen medical suites, each of which resembles a small living room with an exam room and bathroom attached. The physician meets and examines the patient in the suite and will also put the

Impact	Estimated Savings
Improved productivity	$1.86 M
Reduced absenteeism	$0.11 M
Total Estimated Savings	**$1.97 M**

FIGURE 7.1 A tally of health-related productivity savings in the 2007–2008 period of Cisco's "HealthConnections" program. Source: Data from estimates supplied by Cisco, Inc.

patient's electronic medical record up on a screen for both to view and discuss. The idea behind this arrangement is that Cisco's beneficiaries do not lose time sitting around in a general waiting area. The time spent with the physician is maximized, and the patient is unlikely to bump into fellow colleagues because he or she is almost immediately escorted to one of the many examination suites. The setup also allows physicians to maximize the time spent discussing any important health issues with the patients. Typically, appointments are scheduled for time slots lasting either twenty-five or fifty-five minutes, far longer than most patients typically have with their physicians in a single visit.

When we spoke to Dr. Hymel in the spring of 2009, employees were not initially seeing cost reductions in their co-pays or in their deductible. Instead, Dr. Hymel notes that Cisco intends to lure its beneficiaries to switch from their regular provider to the on-campus site by offering a convenient and hassle-free experience, rather than by initially offering monetary savings. She emphasized that in the future, providing the on-campus health care services at a lower price may also be an option to add incentive for beneficiaries to leave their current providers. Dr. Hymel indicated that she and others involved in launching the program had felt that offering care at a lower out-of-pocket patient contribution was not necessary in the early days of the program. Co-pays were similar and in keeping with competing and outside providers when the facility opened. This approach has since changed, and a financial incentive has been offered to patients willing to switch from their current provider to the on-campus facility. Finally, Dr. Hymel added, other Cisco campuses would replicate this program and investment. She also said that Cisco was even looking to provide something analogous to the facility and related programs on its campuses overseas. Cisco has just opened a clinic on its campus in Bangalore, India.

7.3 CASE VIGNETTE: CISCO'S VALUE PROPOSITION— EVALUATING THE REGIONAL, NATIONAL, AND GLOBAL IMPLICATIONS

Before ever discussing this case vignette with a classroom full of students or health care professionals, I sat down to contemplate what the local, regional, and national implications were for these business propositions and the stakeholders involved. Cisco is a company willing to invest a great deal of time, effort, and capital into what may be seen by some as classic preventative medicine coupled with improvements to health care access. Certainly, its investment is one that many other companies will be watching closely. Current technology allows Cisco to integrate and approve many new and sensitive tools that look at both overall health care purchasing costs and productivity. Cisco's value proposition is not only about improving the health of its workforce; it is also about managing its overall labor costs. In this regard, the program serves double duty—perhaps providing a healthier, more productive workforce, but also giving Cisco valuable know-how and a leading edge in delivering integrated health solutions. Tools, software, and management skills honed over the course of this program could eventually supply Cisco with a competitive edge on a saleable product. Therefore, considering the investment only as a labor- or beneficiary-related cost-savings measure would be an underestimation of Cisco's expectations.

Cisco rolled out this program at an interesting time—during one of the worst recessions on record in the United States. Many successful companies, including Cisco, have cut staff amid falling sales and profitability (Gonsalves, 2009). Still, the health care investment was viewed by some as a long-term strategy to retain and reinvest in employees. Cisco's human resources department has long maintained a talent-focused approach to acquiring and retaining top performers in the industry, even in tougher economic times (Kiger, 2003). What does the potential patient-consumer/beneficiary think of this investment? I asked one Cisco employee to give his take (anonymously) on his benefits package, and to gauge how his fellow colleagues felt about it. This e-mail correspondence resulted in the question-and-answer session featured in Box 7.1. Of course, this is in no way a definitive survey from Cisco employees. Instead, I wanted to capture here a rough feet-on-the-ground interview, which adds to the discussion in this case vignette.

Apart from speaking to a Cisco employee, I also discussed Cisco's program with a few of my own colleagues and sought their reaction. These colleagues come from different walks of life and backgrounds, and they brought very different ideas to the table. We discussed the stakeholders involved in the case vignette—both those apparent and those that were more hidden. We spoke about what the actions of purchasers mean for other stakeholders. I realized that the picture of stakeholders that emerged was both expected and surprising. In the actions Cisco is taking, there are many stakeholders that share the value of placing a high priority on attaining better health outcomes as a means of lowering costs. For example, there are the many academic and consulting partners involved in launching the program, as well as in-house Cisco management, including Dr. Hymel and her team. Dr. Hymel's team is constantly combing through the cost data, but they are also actively benchmarking morbidity through the outcome and productivity data. Software developers within Cisco may see themselves as separate stakeholding entities in the promise of a "seamless" health care delivery solution. Employees, as patient-consumers, become successful stakeholder partners when they adopt the several measures to improve healthy lifestyles. Insurers are also in alignment with the efforts to lower costs through better health outcomes. (Insurers, however, will still play the traditional role of interfacing with large providers such as local hospitals and regional hospital networks that are outside Cisco's direct control.)

Many other stakeholders play a direct role in Cisco's value proposition, even if they may not be as closely aligned with the stakeholders mentioned above. There are the companies responsible for contracting the medical and professional staff involved in running the on-campus facility. There are also other competing providers such as local primary care and pediatric physicians, specialists, hospitals, free-standing ambulatory centers, and pharmacies. Local governmental bodies and politicians may be involved to varying degrees. Additionally, the landlords providing space for competing health care and health services providers, local developers, and real estate investors may be impacted or interested in the impact of Cisco's

> **Box 7.1** An Interview with a Cisco Employee
>
> *Have you switched from your current doctors to one of the on-campus doctors in the new Life Connections Health Center provided by Cisco?*
>
> "We decided not to switch from our current doctors to the Cisco on-campus physicians. As we live somewhat far away from campus, it really is not convenient in any case for the family except for myself. As for myself, I don't have a need to visit the doctor frequently, so having one on-campus does not make much of a difference. Also, last year when they opened the facility, there was no financial incentive to change as the deductibles and co-pays were the same. This year, they have changed that, with some deductibles being waived at the on-campus facility. Still, the advantage of keeping the same pediatrician for the kids has outweighed the financial benefit for us and we decided this year to stick with our current doctors. I do use the on-campus pharmacy (a Walgreen's). It's convenient to pick up prescriptions there."
>
> *Do you worry about privacy or simply bumping into colleagues while seeking care on campus?*
>
> "I am not particularly bothered by privacy issues at the on-campus facility. Cisco did a good job in addressing these questions by communicating clearly up front that the facility was operated by an independent firm and there would be no privacy violations. Also, it is such a large campus with so many buildings that I would think the chances of bumping into a colleague at the doctor's are pretty small anyway."
>
> *Do you think the effort Cisco has undertaken should also result in cost savings for the employees, as well as for the company itself?*
>
> "Yes. I think both Cisco and the employee should see savings for the on-campus facility to be viable. Even if the costs are the same as outside to Cisco, I think they gain in employee productivity when the on-campus facility is used. They have been advertising this. With the economy of scale, Cisco should be able to negotiate better rates with providers and pass on some of those savings to users. Also, it is an opportunity for Cisco to pilot its own technology/products in this space. For employees, especially ones that already have a primary care provider established, there is the concern with change. To offset this there has to be some savings. Cisco realized that this year when they waived the deductibles [at the on site facility]."

on-campus health facility. After all, there are as many as forty-five thousand Cisco beneficiaries in the San Jose area. The consequences of a large proportion switching from their current primary care and family practitioners could damage the business prospects of some local providers. How these providers decide to compete with Cisco's on-campus facility could influence, in turn, the future of the on-campus facility's success.

I have often reflected on how the physician–patient relationship may change with the different setup. I have also been thinking about how the nontraditional surroundings may affect the behavior of both the doctor and the patient. In Cisco's on-campus model, the two will meet in a room that resembles a living room more than a stark examination unit. Patients are also (perhaps for the first time) seeing their own medical records up on flat screen. Doctors will be entering notes into a laptop, not scribbling them down in a penmanship often decipherable only to themselves. The time allotted for the visit is longer, allowing for greater exchange of information and concerns. The success of the center will surely turn on the employees' comfort level with the on-campus physicians, and their willingness to switch to the on-campus facility if they already have a doctor they know and trust. Patient and physician priorities must be closely aligned for the continuation of patronage and the program's/facility's success.

I asked my colleagues if Cisco's investment would have an impact on health care going forward. One of my colleagues posited that Cisco's strategy is an effort to become more self-sufficient and less vulnerable to trends in health care inflation. We also agreed that the effort may have local and regional influences on companies competing for the same pool of talent in years to come. The fact that Cisco is a large and highly visible corporation suggests that other companies in a similar league may also be able to compete on the health proposition that Cisco offers its employees. The larger strategy here was to become a more profitable company. Yet, if the strategy showed long-term success in the notable improvement of health outcomes and lowered health spending, it would serve as an influential example that competitors may adopt and emulate. I concur with my colleagues that the work and research that Cisco and its stakeholders have undertaken may serve as a powerful illustrative example, not only for private sector competitors but also for health care provision in the public sector.

In contrast, another colleague argued that even companies as big and as powerful as Cisco would likely have little influence over rising health care costs locally, regionally, or nationally. In the most cynical of scenarios, Cisco would gain vital experience and knowledge about how to improve worker productivity, overall health, and spending on beneficiaries, but would eventually look to move the model overseas (where it might be cheaper to implement and sustain) while rolling back coverage and spending on U.S. campuses. This colleague cited the fact that Cisco intended to roll out a similar health care program with a medical home in India—a place where the program's return on investment might be even greater. I duly note these comments, but I believe that a corporate strategy to invest more specifically in promoting better health outcomes on a small scale (like an office campus) here in the United States can have a large and very positive influence regionally and nationally. In the next section we outline how health care stakeholders may influence each area of the value creation process proposed by proponents of Lean thinking.

7.4 HOW CAN WE IDENTIFY THE VALUE CREATION PROCESS IN HEALTH CARE?

In this chapter, we have covered a lot of ground about how different purchasers have endeavored to hold down health-related expenses while purchasing health care access for their beneficiaries. A close read of this chapter reveals that something quite dynamic is happening among different purchasers and purchaser communities.

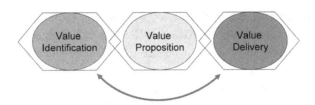

FIGURE 7.2 A model for value creation proposed by Professor Murman and colleagues. Adapted from Figure 1.2 p. 11 in Lean enterprise value: Insights from MIT's lean aerospace initiative by E. Murman, T. Allen, K. Bozdogan, J. Cutcher-Gershenfeld, H. McManus, D. Nightingale, et al., 2002, p. 11. Adapted with permission from Palgrave Macmillan.

To better understand how different stakeholders may fit into the health care value proposition of offering higher-quality, more cost-effective care, we want to introduce a model proposed by Professor Murman and colleagues, which is displayed in Figure 7.2.

Cisco's value proposition among its fellow stakeholders is one that has many aspects and possible areas for value creation. On the surface, the company's investment may appear to be mostly concerned with holding down costs in a market where health care provision is unstoppably inflationary. Therefore, a great part of the value proposition of providing better, higher-touch care is that disease, and the costs associated with unchecked morbidity, will be mitigated by preventative medicine. But this is only one small part of the value proposition. The second, less obvious goal is that healthier workers will, over time, prove to be better, more productive workers. A third major goal for Cisco specifically may be that there are (yet-to-be-known, unquantifiable) gains made in the development of tools, software, and know-how from rolling out several health-solutions-related products, even if some only ever see internal use. To relate this back to Professor Murman's model, we ask a simple question: what value is gained through the value-creation process, and how? This is not a question that can be answered in one phrase or sentence, or even in a single paragraph. The idea behind using this model is to constantly review the expectations of the major stakeholders as the value-creation process evolves and as the goals of the process unfold and mature. This is also the best way to ensure that stakeholders' goals may remain in alignment going forward.

For example, a company may start with a very meager health-enhancement program and then see some savings in terms of health spending on beneficiaries. It may decide to recruit more stakeholders into the process and invest more readily in beneficiaries' health and well-being. Initially, the company's management may have a single goal of containing spending on health benefits through better preventative care, but these ideas may evolve to include goals of higher work productivity and gaining competitive advantage. We adopted the model in Figure 7.2 because, like Professor Murman, we are also emphasizing the possibility that even good efforts toward creating value may be piecemeal in nature, especially in the early stages of a project. In Chapter 8 we draw together the vast literature and experience on stakeholder theory and discuss how we may seek alignment and ultimately greater, lasting value in the health care environment.

REFERENCES

Burton, W. N., Chen, C. Y., Conti, D. J., Schultz, A. B., & Edington, D. W. (2003). Measuring the relationship between employees' health risk factors and corporate pharmaceutical expenditures. *Journal of Occupational and Environmental Medicine, 45*(8), 793–802.

Burton, W. N., Morrison, A., & Wertheimer, A. I. (2003). Pharmaceuticals and worker productivity loss: A critical review of the literature. *Journal of Occupational and Environmental Medicine, 45*(6), 610–621.

Goetzel, R. Z., Long, S. R., Ozminkowski, R. J., Hawkins, K., Wang, S., & Lynch, W. (2004). Health, absence, disability, and presenteeism cost estimates of certain physical and mental health conditions affecting U.S. employers. *Journal of Occupational and Environmental Medicine, 46*(4), 398–412.

Gonsalves, A. (2009, July 16). Cisco lays off hundreds of workers. *InformationWeek*.

Harvard School of Medicine. (2010). Cisco Systems Inc. employee health outreach program. Retrieved January 26, 2010, from http://www.hcp.med.harvard.edu/hpq/ftpdir/Cisco%20EHOP.pdf

Hemp, P. (2004). Presenteeism: At work—but out of it. *Harvard Business Review, 82*(10), 49–58.

Hilton, M. F., Scuffham, P. A., Sheridan, J., Cleary, C. M., & Whiteford, H. A. (2008). Mental ill-health and the differential effect of employee type on absenteeism and presenteeism. *Journal of Occupational and Environmental Medicine, 50*(11), 1228–1243.

Kessler, R. C., Ames, M., Hymel, P. A., Loeppke, R., McKenas, D. K., Richling, D. E., et al. (2004). Using the World Health Organization Health and Work Performance Questionnaire (HPQ) to evaluate the indirect workplace costs of illness. *Journal of Occupational and Environmental Medicine, 46*(6 Suppl), S23–S37.

Kiger, P. J. (2003). Cisco's homegrown gamble. *Workforce, March*, 34.

Loeppke, R., Taitel, M., Haufle, V., Parry, T., Kessler, R. C., & Jinnett, K. (2009). Health and productivity as a business strategy: A multiemployer study. *Journal of Occupational and Environmental Medicine, 51*(4), 411–428.

Loeppke, R., Taitel, M., Richling, D., Parry, T., Kessler, R. C., Hymel, P., et al. (2007). Health and productivity as a business strategy. *Journal of Occupational and Environmental Medicine, 49*(7), 712–721.

Mahoney, J., & Hom, D. (2006). *Total value total return: Seven rules for optimizing employee health benefits for a healthier and more productive workforce*. Philadephia: GlaxoSmithKline.

Murman, E., Allen, T., Bozdogan, K., Cutcher-Gershenfeld, J., McManus, H., Nightingale, D., et al. (2002). *Lean enterprise value: Insights from MIT's lean aerospace initiative*. New York: Palgrave.

Sia, C., Tonniges, T. F., Osterhus, E., & Taba, S. (2004). History of the medical home concept. *Pediatrics, 113*(5 Suppl), 1473–1478.

Wang, P. S., Beck, A., Berglund, P., Leutzinger, J. A., Pronk, N., Richling, D., et al. (2003). Chronic medical conditions and work performance in the Health and Work Performance Questionnaire calibration surveys. *Journal of Occupational and Environmental Medicine, 45*(12), 1303–1311.

8 Fry or Jump: Health Care Stakeholders and the Triggers for Change

8.1 STANDING ON A BURNING PLATFORM

On a summer evening in 1988, an oil-drilling platform off the coast of Scotland caught fire after several explosions (British Broadcasting Corporation [BBC], 2004a, 2004b). The blasts and the inferno that followed were so intense that the platform quickly broke into disconnected pieces. Parts of the platform were incinerated almost immediately by the explosions, and a portion of the platform broke away and fell into the ocean (Smith, Constable, & Gibson, 1988). Crew members who survived the initial explosions quickly found that all the conventional escape routes had been engulfed in flames, so many of them made their way to the platform's edge.

Among these crew members was Andy Mochan, who worked as a superintendent on the oil rig (Smith et al., 1988). As he peered over the platform's edge, he weighed his prospects for survival. He knew that the impact from jumping 150 feet could kill him as he hit the water below. He also knew that the icy waters could be just as deadly as a fire—and even if he did survive the drop and the freezing temperatures, the ocean's surface was littered with debris and burning oil, posing yet another deadly hazard. Despite this, Mr. Mochan jumped, and survived to tell of the horror. Later, when interviewed by reporters, he said that his decision was simple: it was to either "fry or jump, so I jumped" (Conner, 1992; Smith et al., 1988). Many crew members perished that night, and only a handful survived. Out of the 227 workers, 166 never made it home alive. Mr. Mochan was one of the few survivors.

A few years later, business writer Daryl Conner used Mr. Mochan's experience as an analogy to be shared with readers of his book *Managing at the Speed of Change: How Resilient Managers Succeed and Prosper* (Conner, 1992). Conner put it this way: Mr. Mochan made a decision based on "possible death over certain death." To paraphrase Conner, Mochan did not choose to jump because he knew he would survive, or for any reason other than that he had no option but to take his chances. And so the analogy of the "burning platform" in business parlance was born. It is one that has translated to businesses across many industries, and it is one that I like to use when discussing the dire straights in which health care stakeholders often find themselves. For purchasers, payers, hospitals, doctors, clinics, government-sponsored health programs, and the many other stakeholders, there is a point during which they face total disaster if they are not willing to take a huge leap forward instead of standing their ground in an environment of change.

So, what are the triggers for change among health care stakeholders? I pose this question frequently. Certainly from a macro-level point of view, stakeholders in health care pursue many types of change through a variety of ongoing internal reforms. Most often, major change is foisted upon health care stakeholders through market trends, the economy, changing demographics, technology (treatment and diagnostic improvements), government regulation, and evolving competition.

In Chapter 2, we reviewed the trend toward increasing costs and the stagnant or decreasing level of health outcomes. To recap: despite improved technology, medicines, and knowledge, the actual health outcomes in the United States have not improved, or have improved very little. More worrying still is that certain populations in the United States appear in some cases to be falling behind populations in the developed world with regard to morbidity and mortality. Part of the problem relates to access to regular preventative health care. Another part of the problem involves the changing demographics in the United States—more aging people are relying on lower-paying publicly funded health plans, and fewer young, healthy people have been injecting cash into the private-sector system of health coverage. These are issues that national health reform legislation will confront for sometime in the future.

These are well-known problems. For this book, we have brought attention to another major problem. These arise from stakeholders being unwilling or unable to form partnerships with one another in order to create lasting value. While the word "partner" might conjure the notion of coupling, we will devote more time to describing multilateral alignments, and not simple bilateral agreements, to move change forward. We need to stress that this is the type of change that cannot be created by legislation or other means of mandated intervention. The triggers of major changes come very often from external forces. In this final chapter, we make the case to begin change from within. Entities that operate in health care need to inform other health care stakeholders and incorporate them into their core operations.

8.2 PUTTING STAKEHOLDER THEORY INTO PERSPECTIVE

So far, we have written, firstly, about a need for stakeholding parties in health care to identify their fellow stakeholders. Secondly, we have mentioned how the stakeholders, and the information that they rely on, tend to get caught in silos that preclude cooperation and alignment. Thirdly, we have written about the barriers to stakeholder alignment that derive from pursuing a customer-centric model of health care delivery. In the world of health care stakeholders, putting the customer "in the center" is not only confusing; it may also be counterproductive. This is the case because a "customer" is ill-defined within health care. Health care consumers could be patients, purchasers of medical goods, nongovernmental sponsors, corporations purchasing group plans, or government-affiliated entities. In health care, the lines between the producer, supplier, vendor, and consumer blur to the point that conventional business models are not terribly useful.

Consider the stakeholder that we commonly refer to as the "patient," or even the more contemporary label, "patient-customer." Many people assume that the patient serves primarily as the consumer of health care, when in reality the patient is also an important supplier or producer of health outcomes. A physician does not only supply treatments to patients; he or she is also a co-producer of health outcomes. An insurer may act on behalf of a corporation to purchase treatments and preventative care; yet by this same reasoning the insurer is also a producer of health outcomes, because this stakeholder plays a role in enforcing quality standards in hospitals and among other providers such as physician practices. Herein we find the major reasons for adopting stakeholder theory instead of traditional business models that rely heavily on identifying suppliers and competitors within an industry; these labels come up short when charting the various health care stakeholders.

Many common business models borrow, explicitly or implicitly, from my colleague Michael Porter's (1985) seminal work *Competitive Advantage: Creating and Sustaining Superior Performance*. This book introduced the concept of value-chain analysis, which posits a series of activities that can add value to a particular product. Porter's value chain has worked extremely well for many industries and has spurred much debate and literature addressing how value accrues through the steps taken to create a final product. A simple example of this accreted product value is the transformation of a diamond in the rough to a cut stone that may be sold at a much higher price; each party's actions, from the miner to the final store manager, create additional value for the person who makes the final purchase.

The value-chain model places the firm (or corporate entity) at the center of value creation. With that business as the locus of activity, Professor Porter also proposed that there are five major forces influencing management strategy. The first force acts through the needs and decisions made by customers. The second force is found in product or service substitutes that threaten existing business. The leverage that suppliers have on a firm's business (through negotiation) count as a third force. The threats posed by new entrants into the market and by the rivalry that already exists between a firm and its close competitors pose a fourth and a fifth force. In Figure 8.1, we can see a schematic representation of these five forces, adapted from Professor Porter's original sketch.

However, since its initial appearance in 1985, this approach has spurred numerous business writers to think of other important forces or entities that exert force on a company—influences such as government.

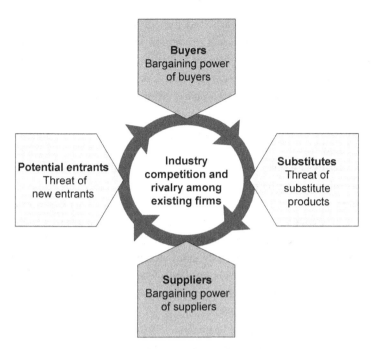

FIGURE 8.1 Porter's five forces shaping industry competition. Adapted from "The Five Forces that Determine Industry Profitability," by M. Porter, 1985, *Competitive advantage: Creating and sustaining superior performance*, p 5. Copyright 1985 by Michael Porter.

In contrast to Porter's models, stakeholder theorist Edward Freeman and his colleagues (2007) argued that putting management or even the customer at the center of any business model is problematic, particularly because it focuses too much attention inward. Recall our review of Professor Freeman's thinking on the managerial-centric approach in Chapter 4; he described how managerial models fail to yield strategies that combine ethics and values. Freeman also contends that the process of value creation should be measured by ethical and other nonfinancial values. He writes of adopting a "stakeholder mindset" and calls for stakeholders to pursue an "enterprise strategy". This thinking has garnered considerable support in recent years. But how can we apply it to the contemporary context of our health care environment?

From our case vignettes, we can see that stakeholder theory, or some semblance of stakeholder theory, has already taken root in industries and activities across the nation. The case vignette in Chapter 7 reveals steps that Cisco Systems made in order to improve the health outcomes of its workforce. The company partnered with several other firms to bring primary care providers to its work sites. It has also strove to engage its employees to better controlling their health by taking advantage of initiatives to improve the management of health problems, through better diet, exercise, and far-reaching initiatives that encourage mental well-being.

Cisco invested extensively in partnerships that bring preventative medicine into its health purchasing plans. Make no mistake, one major driver behind this effort is cost savings. The cost savings are found most concretely in purchasing care for its beneficiaries, but they are also achieved through higher employee productivity during the workday. These efforts will, in addition, improve the quality of life for its employees and the beneficiaries' families. In this manner, these goals represent part of Cisco's ethical responsibility to its workforce. Taking on this ethical responsibility has since had a major ripple effect. Cisco has invested in quality care for its employees in Bangalore, India, where health interventions may have a major impact on quality of living. This ripple effect will not stop with Cisco, as other corporations are likely to follow suit.

Other health care stakeholders have looked to the philosophy and principles of Lean thinking to bring better value to their operations. Lean thinking and stakeholder theory are natural complements as far as business strategy is concerned. As noted in earlier chapters, the philosophy which eventually evolved into Lean thinking emerged from the Toyota Production System of Taiichi Ohno (1988). In some aspects, Professor Freeman was likely influenced by Mr. Ohno's thinking. This is because Mr. Ohno promoted the idea of always seeing Toyota's parts suppliers, vendors, and customers as stakeholders in the company's pledge of building a product of unparalleled quality (Ohno, 1988).

However, as we put thoughts to paper in mid-2010, we found it more than ironic that Toyota was facing scandals involving the safety and reliability of its vehicles. In trying to correct these major problems and regain the trust of its customers and the government, the management at Toyota hinted that it would return to the original thinking of Mr. Ohno. In an appearance before the U.S. House Oversight and Government Reform Committee, the company's president, Akio Toyoda (the grandson of the company's founder), acknowledged: "I fear the pace at which we have grown may have been too quick" (Vartabedian & Bensinger, 2010). From his testimony and thoughts, it became clear that his management team had lost sight of their stakeholders as participants in the creation of value. Sadly, his business strategy had evolved from one of stakeholder participation into what Freeman might describe as a managerial-centric model. The range of voices and partnerships narrowed, and the ability to promote novel advantages and ensure the highest quality decreased. This is a good example of an approach that lacks a strong enterprise strategy promoting ethics and values.

As discussed in previous chapters, one major dictate of Lean thinking is to "pull" value from the consumer. In other words, a successful corporation looks to listen to and act on continual feedback from its users (customers) and other stakeholders. Because Toyota's management did not effectively partner with American experts or even its own internal safety experts, serious quality issues went unchecked. As many investigative reports indicated, a culture of secrecy flourished among the managers. The relationships between Toyota and these important stakeholders deteriorated until they became extremely contentious and dysfunctional (Linebaugh, Searcey, & Shirouzu, 2010).

In health care as in the auto industry, there are always those that reduce product or service value, wittingly or not, because they do not partner with their fellow stakeholders. Fortunately, most managers eagerly seek to create value—yet many lack the tools and know-how to do so. This is where the Forces of Change Program fits into the equation. I always make a point of emphasizing that stakeholder theory occupies pole position in the Forces of Change Model. For years, I have been tracking positive and successful health care stories among stakeholders seeking to become more effective in bringing value to health care. The Program's curriculum content and exercises prod participants to produce systematic changes to their operations in order bring greater value to their place in the health care ecology. More importantly, they also learn strategies to transcend contentious standoffs and impasses with real solutions. I have long focused on fostering beneficial cooperation and healthy co-opetition. Now, in this time of complex and uncertain reforms, there has never been as great a moment to take advantage of the changes at hand. In Section 8.3, we talk about identifying agents of positive change, and in the final section of this chapter and book we review recent innovations that have proffered useful tools of change.

8.3 THE ENABLERS: FINDING THOSE THAT CAN FACILITATE ALIGNMENT

There are vast differences between the auto and health care industries, right? (Bear with me; this is yet another exercise in thinking.) For starters, a vehicle is a tangible good, while health care is an intangible service. *Is this correct?* I often ask of my participants. The answer to this question is not as clear as it may seem. This can spark a wonderful debate. The Toyota debacle, which hit the news in the latter part of 2009, highlighted what many business analysts have misunderstood for decades.

Industry stakeholders often do not fully realize what product they are selling to consumers. Over the years, Toyota's management placed such a great priority on the growth in sales of its vehicles that it lost sight of its true value proposition, which is total reliability in safely getting from one place to another. Similarly, many health care stakeholders have lost sight of *their* true value proposition. They may imagine a product of immediate significance instead of one of long-term importance. For example, a private practice may focus so heavily on a new technology for its competitive edge that the doctors in the practice start to see themselves as providers of diagnoses and treatments to their patients; yet these doctors are really in the business of producing improved health outcomes among a patient population.

The doctors in this hypothetical practice may balk at this last statement, saying something like, "We can't control health outcomes, we can only offer treatment and care interventions!" But this thinking, we contend, is outdated. What we am offering is a stakeholder perspective. As a stakeholder in health care, a physician's practice may create greater value by partnering with other stakeholders. A particular practice may team up with other practices, purchasers, insurers, and promoters of wellness to build more-effective care alliances with their patients. They can look to foster a continuum of care that influences health outcomes positively. They need to identify opportunities to align or, at the very least, co-compete with other entities. Together with their multiple and related stakeholders, they can work toward producing better health outcomes and, therefore, value.

We want to also introduce one more component of Toyota's Lean methods—one that was devised by Mr. Ohno himself. This is the concept of the "andon," which is sometimes referred to as the "andon cord" or "andon board." This is not only a concept; it is also a physical tool. It can comprise a hanging cord attached to some sort of alarm for getting attention, or an electronic board with lights that signal the need for different levels of attention and action (Ohno, 1988). The key characteristic of the andon is that it is accessible to all the workers on the factory floor. By triggering the device, the factory worker can get the attention of his or her supervisors and coworkers immediately to resolve a problem as soon as it appears. Yes, this means that the worker pauses or even halts production on a particular product and disrupts the flow of work in the entire process. However, despite seconds or minutes of lost productivity, the benefits of this tool are measurable. This is true because minor flaws in production may be caught and resolved immediately, before they lead to bigger problems that trigger greater downtime in production. Mr. Ohno used this method to eliminate the faulty parts that would result in lengthy productivity delays or, worse, unreliable cars.

In the face of Toyota's 2010 safety scandals, Akio Toyoda, the company's president, under much public and governmental pressure, eventually came forward to personally apologize. He also halted sales and production, and he ordered the recall of thousands of vehicles already in customers' hands. More interesting was his curiously titled open letter to the public: "Toyota's plan to repair its public image" (Toyoda, 2010). In the letter he makes an analogy to demonstrate his commitment to improving the notorious culture of silence that led to the safety problems. Here is an excerpt from his letter, which appeared in the *Washington Post*:

For much of Toyota's history, we have ensured the quality and reliability of our vehicles by placing a device called an andon cord on every production line—and empowering any team member to halt production if there's an assembly problem. Only when the problem is resolved does the line begin to move again. Two weeks ago, I pulled the andon cord for our company.

Mr. Toyoda's words are both telling and inept. Having to make a far-reaching public apology in the face of government pressure, and having to halt production on such a large scale, is a worst-case scenario. The debacle will appear and reappear in business and history books for decades to come. The andon cord is not intended as a tool for the top management to use in a catastrophe. The andon is an everyday tool for the workers on the floor to use to keep quality as a number one priority. It is a tool that empowers all of the workers, making them a stakeholder in the final product. Toyota's problems in 2010 were far greater than a "public image" crisis—they had spiraled into a stakeholder-trust crisis.

To make this example relevant to health care stakeholders, we are advocating two things. Firstly, we are calling on health care stakeholders to build strong alignments with one another. Secondly, health care stakeholders must also improve their communication within their organization to accomplish the first task. The andon can constitute a tool that may help all the many individuals working within a health care entity to keep the focus on safety, affordability, and quality care. A health care andon can take many physical forms, but, importantly, it always serves as a way of sounding the alarm and drawing attention to a problem. If all workers, regardless of their status, have access to the andon, they can immediately see mistakes or inefficiencies when they occur. However, there is more to this thinking than simply empowering employees to better troubleshoot.

Up until this point, we have written mainly about improving alignment through creating open lines of continual communication between stakeholders. We also want to highlight how the many individuals working within every health care stakeholder group must feel that they are themselves stakeholders in the promise of better value. By better value, we mean making a positive impact on health outcomes. One of the major reasons that Professor Freeman conceived of enterprise strategy is because he felt that corporate entities had cleaved pursuing business from pursuing ethical and value-oriented goals (Freeman et al., 2007). He suggests that a stakeholder approach could resolve misdirected strategies and poorly conceived goals.

We are extending Dr. Freeman's thinking a few steps further. He wrote that a business would only work if the different stakeholders influenced by that business "get their needs and desires satisfied, over time" (Freeman et al., 2007). Freeman and we agree that stakeholders cannot force one another into alignment any more than they can simply force their workers to be less prone to mistakes and inefficiencies. Therefore, the stakeholder ethic can only permeate an entity when the individuals themselves hold the stakes. Workers are the potential enablers in a promise for better value, and they are the crucial enablers in the forging of a stakeholder alignment; yet they are only likely to become enablers if they feel a responsibility to cooperate. These potential enablers also need the right tools, and they need to reside in the right environment, if they are to be empowered with a mission of adding greater value. While this section has focused on identifying the potential enablers, we now turn our attention to identifying the tools that allow an entity to transform its traditional outlook into a stakeholder mindset.

8.4 THE CURRENT FORCES OF CHANGE: BETTER TOOLS AND BETTER UTILIZATION OF THESE TOOLS

One day, after lengthy discussion with my colleagues about how and why stakeholders initiate alignment, I noticed that something was missing from our analysis. I began to ask myself and then my colleagues why stakeholders should bother to seek alignment in the first place. Initially, some of my colleagues bristled at the question, shooting me odd looks and answering my question with another question. They would ask something to this effect: "Isn't this what we've been discussing this whole time?" Or they would say: "Health care stakeholders need to seek alignment because they work so closely they have to come to some sort of accommodation of one another's needs." This premise is false; many health care stakeholders have worked closely together for years or even decades without a sense of true alignment. Let us think back to our case vignette involving Thomas Jones, who negotiates reimbursements for his health system with payers and insurers.

It is clear that Jones sometimes negotiates deals where there is little or no accommodation between the payers and the workers within his health care system. Because his health care system is one of the bigger players in that particular market, Mr. Jones is able to approach negotiations with an upper hand, and can secure favorable reimbursements for the staff and hospital visits. In his words—and in the words of some of his colleagues—there is a sense of control and confidence. This control, however, does not extend to all situations.

Our second vignette in Chapter 6 showed how some of the heart specialists who work within Mr. Jones's health system vied for more control over how insurers could employ "appropriateness" criteria. The cardiologists represented some of the best in their field in terms of care and research, and they felt threatened by the prospect of insurers' determining which sequence of tests and diagnoses would be covered. These specialists argued that they could provide more insight into how care is administered, or under which circumstances care would be labeled "inappropriate." To try to assuage the cardiologists' concerns and meet the expectations of an insurer (and the many payers), Mr. Jones developed a narrative about partnering and allowing physicians to self-manage as far as appropriateness criteria are concerned. Unfortunately, the insurer did not buy into this narrative, and so the proposal and that particular discussion failed to produce alignment.

So, what is the take-away from this case vignette? Perhaps the lesson is that good ideas often fail because the different stakeholders are not comfortable with the agreement. Indeed, there are stakeholders who have the capacity to enable change yet, for numerous reasons, cannot convince their fellow stakeholders to join in those changes. We use the expression "institutional memory" to describe this type of inertia that exists within or between stakeholders. To say simply that the various stakeholders lack vision or courage would be disingenuous. The problem, often, is far more complex. Within companies or organizations, an institutional memory connotes a type of narrative among workers and management that is told and retold about a particular experience (Linde, 2009). When this narrative is about a failure, it can influence future attempts at success. This may mean that there are extensive scars from past, failed, or unfinished attempts at alignment. The stakeholders and the people working within a stakeholder group may see alignment with one or more fellow stakeholders as a Sisyphean task, and therefore avoid any changes in thinking or processes that allow alignment.

In talking with and working alongside health care leaders for a quarter of a century, I have seen clearly that the resistance to instituting changes springs from past disappointments. Therefore, I often urge my participants to focus first on small and seemingly inconsequential opportunities that exist going forward, simply to initiate a sort of momentum. I find that when I am working with a health care organization to increase efficiency, the managers tend to complain that they lack the resources or the talent needed to improve their operation. But it is at this point that I remind them of a contemporary phenomenon commonly referred to as "Joy's Law," after Bill Joy, the cofounder of Sun Microsystems. According to some accounts, he openly posited that "no matter who you are, most of the smartest people work for someone else" (Lakhani & Panetta, 2007). This view may seem particularly bleak.

However, Mr. Joy was not hinting at a crisis in human resources; instead, his words foreshadowed a new wave of innovation.

Joy's comment marked the proliferation of shared innovation, the kind of innovation that produced the open-source software (OSS) movement over the past twenty years. While this movement has its roots in free-software distributive efforts of the 1980s, OSS took off as the Internet expanded. OSS is developed in the public domain by the very users it serves. Mr. Joy's words are often repeated with a view that all sorts of open innovation have been made possible through technological advances and changes in thinking. Because the people developing the OSS typically represent volunteers who want to use the software for their own benefit, the process is at its core user-driven (Lakhani & Panetta, 2007).

In an open innovation initiative, many minds drive the production of a product—a product that will likely evolve to be stronger and more reliable than one designed by a single company. Economist Eric von Hippel detailed the concept and benefits of distributed innovation in his 2005 book. In this work, he explains that traditionally, a single company or organization designs a service or product to satisfy its perception of user needs. This customary mode of innovation is closed and does not take advantage of successful ideas that come from the users themselves (von Hippel, 2005). Now, in many industries, there is a shift toward embracing distributed innovation. This trend is emerging despite the fact that many companies stayed away from multisource innovation for so many years, fearing that it would invite complications, covert competition, or copyright infringement and privacy concerns. Indeed, the shift toward open innovation mimics the concept of "pull" from Lean manufacturing, detailed in previous chapters. The idea is to follow the users closely and better understand their desires and needs, and thus to "pull" value directly from the user experience. Once a design fully incorporates root sources of feedback from users, the final product can carry much more value.

I want to circle back to an example of how distributed innovation is at the forefront of improvement. A service or product may be designed with good intentions, and with the best materials, expertise, and care. However, even if designers simply study the users, many of the wants and needs can get "lost in translation," so to speak. When this happens, the likelihood of designing a quality product declines. Therefore, I have long embraced the notion of defining "quality" by the products' and services' fitness for use. In other words, a product or service may not be high quality unless it fulfills the needs of the user. No one can really understand the user's needs except for the user himself or herself. So why not have the user design the product? This is the concept at the heart of user-generated distributed innovation.

Today, many large and small corporations and organizations are tapping into the benefits of user-designed or user-modified products and services. They are doing this with the help of specialized software and strategies that allow users to customize services and products to their liking. This user-led movement is a major driver for change in today's business world. Despite this, the health care world has done little in this area of innovation.

Applying the user-led techniques may be challenging, but *not* anticipating the need to make use of distributed knowledge is even more perilous. In Chapter 4, we reviewed the concept of silos and noted how knowledge and expertise get stuck in these isolated towers. Some thinkers contend that innovative knowledge, by its very nature, is "sticky" (von Hippel, 1994). New ideas, when clearly articulated so that their advantages are readily apparent, have the power to change stakeholder patterns of behavior and overcome the inertia produced by institutional memories. This is precisely why I tell my colleagues that the challenge does not lie in identifying areas needing improvement because communication is poor or alignment is nonexistent; the challenge instead is in extracting knowledge and distributing the expertise to benefit all stakeholders. This is a topic that I address in great depth during my Forces of Change Executive Programs.

Recently I came across a strong and intriguing example of how a number of companies are trying to use open innovation to break down knowledge silos and reduce their carbon footprint. The leader in this particular effort is the sportswear brand Nike. The company has sought to reduce its carbon footprint by modifying its supply chains, manufacturing processes, logistics, communications, and technology use (Shahan, 2010). This reduction of the carbon footprint was not attributable to the recent economic slowdown or to cutbacks in business and sales. To the contrary, the sporting-goods giant reported revenue growth while making steady improvements in reducing carbon footprint. By using a particular open-innovation tool, Nike demonstrated its intention to share its homegrown knowledge with others looking to make equivalent or similar improvements. Nike entered into a deal to participate in a Web-based marketplace called GreenXchange, or GX. When this new alignment was announced in early 2010 at the World Economic Forum in Davos, Switzerland, nine other entities agreed to participate. Some of the corporations are large commercial organizations, such Best Buy and salesforce.com; others are nonprofits, such as Creative Commons (Shahan, 2010). Yet all of these stakeholders share the commitment of reducing both the cost and the environmental impact of doing business. They act according to a shared expectation and have come to alignment on the direction of their expectation.

This effort will likely harvest a crop of very successful innovations, because the exchange has been set up to capture ideas from a crowd. Indeed, the use of open, user-generated innovation often carries the moniker of "crowdsourcing" or community-based design (Malone, Laubacher, & Dellarocas, 2010) because it involves a group of people that may or may not be easily defined. Historically, entities shy away from using tools that rely on a crowd because it may seem too unfocused as an idea generator. However, recently researchers at MIT have defined ways of productively focusing the power of innovative crowds (Malone et al., 2010). One MIT research group in particular has built a model to encourage a collective intelligence system that is strongly goal specific (see Figure 8.2).

Through this model, we can see that collective intelligence does not have to be something that appears serendipitously, as did the organic evolution of OSS. Collective intelligence can be cultivated, harvested, and customized. Nike and its stakeholders have already discovered this for themselves.

In this book, we have devoted several chapters to introducing and examining the idea of aligned expectations among stakeholders. One common exercise used by

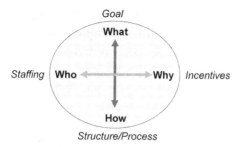

FIGURE 8.2 Collective intelligence: what are the four main questions? Adapted from "The collective intelligence genome," by T.W. Malone, R. Laubacher, & C. Dellarocas, 2010, *MIT Sloan Management Review, 51*, p 23. Copyright 2010 by Massachusetts Institute of Technology. All rights reserved. Distributed by Tribune Media Services.

past writers on stakeholder theory in health care proposes making lists of all the stakeholders involved in any given situation (Blair & Fottler, 1990). However, the construction of lists is but a first step. We take this type of analysis many paces further. We prefer to list the stakeholders in every area of the value-creation process and then determine whether some stakeholders are missing or excluded from one area. If they are, we study whether they may be persuaded or invited to participate in the other areas. Additionally, I ask small crowds (like a classroom full of executive participants) to try to inhabit one or more stakeholder mindsets for the purposes of a case study. These imagined groups then prioritize a list of must-do items. The exercise can provide a snapshot of how far apart or how closely aligned the stakeholders may feel in any given situation. Charting the distance between stakeholders, and the entrenchment of the causes of this distancing, represents just one of many tools we have that help entities to move toward greater alignment, efficiency, and, ultimately, increased value potential.

8.5 THE COMMONS AND HEALTH CARE IN A CONTEMPORARY CONTEXT

We opened this chapter by writing about the concept of burning platforms, but as of yet, we have said little about the burning platforms in health care. Certainly, burning platforms do seem to surround us—many purchasers are either straining under the rising costs of healthcare or deciding to exit the game all together. Yet some purchasers, like Cisco, have decided to jump. They are swimming in the other direction, toward making larger and longer-term investments in the health of their beneficiaries. These companies are doing this perhaps because their leaders understand that human talent is at the core of their own value proposition. Cisco, a major player in the technology industry, with peers such as Google, Intel, Apple, and Oracle, faces a perpetual burning platform. Nonetheless, they are among a group of health purchasers that expend a constant effort to produce the next new technology, the new direction or the new big idea that will allow them to do business going forward. If these companies see their employees as their most valuable asset, they might be motivated to make substantial investments in keeping their talent. In contrast, purchasers in other, older industries may not see themselves as standing on a burning platform because they occupy a space that appears safe from established competition. Such feelings of comfortable isolation are, however, chimerical, as all major industries face the challenge of managing the inflationary costs of health care, and of getting ideal productivity out of their employees.

It is easy to see how health care stakeholders stand on perpetually burning platforms. The many different types of providers are racing about on the burning platform, caught between the high operating costs and the need to compete for a diminishing pool of privately funded patients. (Clark, 2009) Insurers, like providers, find themselves on equally fiery footing. New federal legislation will likely force private payers to provide coverage for a much wider pool of beneficiaries. No doubt, this will require major changes to their way of doing business. Furthermore, changes within the insurance industry will have a major ripple effect on providers, patients, and purchasers. Currently, the patient population faces ever-encroaching flames. More and more patients face serious but preventable or treatable health conditions, yet they are not empowered to get treatment or take control of their problems. All these burning platforms carry wide-ranging implications that beg for stark and immediate change.

Change, however, requires problem-solving tools capable of drawing upon adequate and innovative knowledge. Here we circle back to the problem of "sticky" information. Professor Eric Von Hippel (1994) of the Sloan School of Management put it this way: "to solve a problem, needed information and problem-solving capabilities must be brought together—physically or *virtually*—at a single locus." And here is the crux of the problem that health care stakeholders face going forward. At present, many stakeholders lack consistent, reliable, and usable information. This is perhaps due to a dearth of transparency, a lack of accurate data, or an inability to harness data in a useful manner—all of which are inherent in our health care culture. Once information has been freed from the silos that exist within every stakeholder in health care, the task of matching information and problem-solving tools will become easier, with resulting gains in efficiency and productivity.

Finally, we return to the analogy of Hardin's (1968) cattle herders, which we used at the beginning of this book. In this analogy, the stakeholders are the "cattle herders" and they compete for dominant access over the shared resource, which is the "land." But we should ask what constitutes "the pasture" when we talk about health care. Some may posit that it is the amount of goodwill that exists among stakeholders. Others may say it is the patient population. Indeed, we would also argue that for health care, the raw resource is the patient, and the product is the patient outcome.

Earlier, we said that the patient was a producer of health outcomes, and we stand by this idea. To follow through with Hardin's analogy, the pasture is an independent factor that influences the cattle's ability to fatten up, regardless of how the cattle or their herders conduct themselves. Extreme weather, be it drought or too much rain, is one of the many factors that will influence the pasture's ability to thrive, the cattle's ability to graze, and, eventually, the herders' well-being. To clarify further, we are suggesting that the patient is a type of herder (producer) and the patient population is the raw material (the resource). Sadly, Hardin's metaphor predicts disaster for the pasture and, eventually, for all the pasture's stakeholders. Yet we are not willing to predict disaster for patient populations and for all of the varied stakeholders in the health care environment.

As Professor Elinor Ostrom, winner of the 2009 Nobel Memorial Prize in Economic Science, observed, we may be obsessed with a few portions of Hardin's "Tragedy of the Commons." In particular, some of us may be seduced by Hardin's metaphor that all users of a common resource are likely to produce suboptimal outcomes unless they are regulated by a centralized authority (Ostrom, 1990). The need for an authority figure hangs as a subtext in Hardin's work because without someone enforcing fairness, there is "tragedy." Luckily, Professor Ostrom challenged this view with her research and writings. In her groundbreaking work *Governing the Commons: The Evolution of Institutions for Collective Action*, Ostrom (1990) argues that there are a number of different solutions for protecting a vital and common resource. For starters, she cites examples of both successful and unsuccessful efforts to escape tragedy when cooperating or co-competing for a common resource. From these illustrations, she is able to outline strategies for parties to manage dire depletions without slipping into catastrophe. Furthermore, Professor Ostrom cautions that reliance on a centralized authority to ensure cooperation often fails because a central authority may never have a full appreciation of the information that lies distributed among the stakeholders. Managing the crisis, therefore, is more likely to be successful if measures are predicated on the knowledge and actions of individual stakeholders rather than controlling bodies.

We want to leave the reader with this final thought: stakeholder success in the health care environment will not depend solely on outside forces of change. By this, we mean that we cannot look solely to overarching proposals involving regulations, government interventions, economic trends, consumerism, or even new medical breakthroughs. Instead, success will lay in the health care stakeholders' ability to self-manage the forces of change from the inside and among their peers. Success will rely on the ability of stakeholders to align themselves with one another to protect the commons that is patient health if good patient outcomes are to be sustainable for years and decades to come.

REFERENCES

Blair, J. D., & Fottler, M. D. (1990). *Challenges in health care management: Strategic perspectives for managing key stakeholders* (1st ed). San Francisco: Jossey-Bass.

British Broadcasting Corporation. (2004a). 1988: Disaster in the North Sea. Retrieved April 19, 2010, from http://news.bbc.co.uk/onthisday/hi/witness/july/6/newsid_3036000/3036510.stm

British Broadcasting Corporation. (2004b). Vivid memories of Piper Alpha. Retrieved April 19, 2010, from http://news.bbc.co.uk/2/hi/uk_news/scotland/3873113.stm

Clarke, R. L. (2009). *Beyond the burning platform: Value strategies for the long term* (Annual Report). Westchester, IL: Healthcare Financial Management Association.

Conner, D. R. (1992). The process of change. In *Managing at the speed of change: How resilient managers succeed and prosper where others fail* (p. 282). New York: Villard Books/Random House.

Freeman, R. E., Harrison, J. S., & Wicks, A. C. (2007). Managing for stakeholders. In *Managing for stakeholders: Survival, reputation and success* (pp. 1–19). New Haven, CT: Yale University Press.

Hardin, G. (1968). The tragedy of the commons. *Science, 162*(5364), 1243–1248.

Lakhani, K. R., & Panetta, J. A. (2007). *The principles of distributed innovation.* Cambridge, MA: The Berkman Center for Internet & Society at Harvard Law School.

Linde, C. (2009). *Working the past: Narrative and institutional memory.* New York: Oxford University Press.

Linebaugh, K., Searcey, D., & Shirouzu, N. (2010, February 8). Secretive culture led Toyota astray. *Wall Street Journal.*

Malone, T. W., Laubacher, R., & Dellarocas, C. (2010). The collective intelligence genome. *MIT Sloan Management Review, 51*(3), 21–31.

Ohno, T. (1988). *Toyota production system: Beyond large-scale production.* New York: Productivity Press.

Ostrom, E. (1990). *Governing the commons: The evolution of institutions for collective action.* Cambridge, UK: Cambridge University Press.

Porter, M. (1985). *Competitive advantage: Creating and sustaining superior performance.* New York: The Free Press, Collier Macmillen.

Shahan, Z. (2010, January 28). Nike cuts carbon footprint, launches sustainability exchange. Matter Network Web site. Retrieved December 2, 2010, from http://www.matter network.com/2010/1/nike-cuts-carbon-footprint-launches.cfm

Smith, W. E., Constable, A., & Gibson, H. (1988, July 18). Disaster screaming like a banshee: An exploding platform takes 166 lives in the North Sea. *Time.*

Toyoda, A. (2010, February 9). Toyota's plan to repair its public image. *Washington Post.*

Vartabedian, R., & Bensinger, K. (2010, February 24). Toyota president Akio Toyoda apologizes for safety lapses. *Los Angeles Times.*

von Hippel, E. (1994). Sticky information and the locus of problem solving. *Management Science, 40*(4), 429–439.

von Hippel, E. (2005). *Democratizing innovation.* Cambridge, MA: MIT Press.

Index

Note: Page numbers followed by "*f*" indicate illustrative figures.

Administrative costs, 27
Aetna, 60–61
Aging population, 22
Agle, Bradley, R., 84–85
Alignment, financial, 80. *See also* stakeholder alignment
Ambulatory surgeries, 81–82
American Society of Echocardiography (ASE), 102
Amico, Russell, 90
Appropriateness criteria, 95–100, 134
Appropriate use, health care services, 71, 75, 89, 99
Assurance practice, 71
Asthma, 25

Baby boomers, 22
Bankruptcy/debt, 43
Banner Health, 61
Benchmarks, of healthcare, 18
Blue Cross Blue Shield of Massachusetts (BCBSMA), 31–32
Boress, Larry, 114
Breast cancer treatment, 29–30, 41–42
"Burning platform" analogy, 126, 137–138

Capitalism, 11–12
Cardiac care, 90–92, 95–99, 100–103
Care coordination, 45, 47
CareCore National, 90
Case basis payments, 80. *See also* reimbursements
"Cattle herding" analogy, 9, 138–139
Centers for Disease Control and Prevention (CDC), 42
Centers for Medicare & Medicaid Services (CMS), 60, 102
Chronic illnesses, 24–25

Churning, 46
Cisco Systems, 117–123, 124, 129–130
Clinton health reforms, 50
Collective intelligence, 136, 137*f*
Commercial payers, 23
Common resource, sharing of, 8, 108
Competition model, 129*f*
Competitors, cross-marketing of, 3
Concierge care, 47–48
Conflict, stakeholder, 71
Consensus building, 6
Consumers, of health care services, 24–25, 28, 60, 65, 69–70, 89
"Co-opetition," 3–4, 11, 13
Cortese, Denis A., 64
Costs
  as cause of conflict, 31–33
  drivers/inflators of, 22–28
  of pharmaceutical drugs, 29–31
  price/rate controls, 79
  technological advances and, 28–31
  of treatment/diagnostics, 50
Cost savings. *See* employer cost savings
"Cost-shift payment hydraulic," 23
Cross-marketing, by competitors, 3
CT scans, overuse of, 71, 90–92, 100–102
Customers, sharing of, 3

Darrow, Greg, 89
"Dartmouth Data," 101, 103
Debt and bankruptcy, 43
Defensive medicine, 29, 71, 89
Delbanco, Tom, 68
Dependency Structure Matrix (DSM), 93
Diabetes, type 2, 24, 49
Disproportionate-share hospital (DSH) program, 24
Distributed innovation, 135–136

Doctors. *See* physicians/doctors
Drugs, new vs. older, 29–31

Emergency department (ED) crowding, 26–27
Employer cost savings, 113–115, 117–123, 124, 129–130
Employer-sponsored health insurance, 22–23, 26, 40–42, 45–47, 49, 113–116
Entitlement model, 22–23
Expectations about health
  access problems and, 42–48
  among stakeholder groups, 41–42
  genetic testing and, 42
  as human right/responsibility, 39–40
  uninsurance and, 42–43
  wellness programs, 49–50
Expenditures on health care, 20, 21f

Federal-type business approach, 5–6
Food and Drug Administration (FDA), 42
Forces of Change Program, 130–131, 136
"Four Ps" (stakeholder groups), 13
France, 18, 20, 21
Free clinics, 44–45
Freeman, Edward R., 10–11, 69–71, 84, 104–105, 129, 133
Friedman, Milton, 11

Game theory, 9
Gawande, Atul, 77
Generic drugs, 29–30
Genetic testing, 41–42
Germany, 18, 20, 21
Goals, alignment of, 4–5
Gordian knot analogy, 32–33
Government Accountability Office (GAO), 29
Government-sponsored health insurance, 23, 45, 50
Grayson, Mary, 6–7
Grossi, Ignacio, 93, 105
Guilmette, Dave, 116

Hardin, Garrett, 8, 9, 108, 138–139
"Harry and Louise" advertising campaign, 50–51

Health care, as human right/responsibility, 39–40
Health Care and Education Reconciliation Act of 2010, 14, 33, 46, 50, 74
Health care community
  as "bickering family," 6–7, 13–14
  coordination efforts, 14
Health care reform, history of, 52
Health outcomes
  access problems, 42–48
  among U.S. peers, 18
  expenditures on, 20, 21f
  indicators of, 19
  stakeholder alignment in, 4
Herzlinger, Regina, 17, 75
Higgins, Michaela J., 41
High-cost-low-quality paradigm, 8–9
Himmelstein, David, 27
Hospital beds, per capita, 21
Hospitals, 62–63, 67–68, 79–80
Hymel, Pamela, 117–121

Imaging utilization, 29, 97–98, 100–101
Impotency drugs, 40–41
Inappropriate testing, 95–100
Indicators, of health, 19
Infant mortality rate, 19
Innovation, distributed, 135–136
Inpatient admissions/services, 81–82
Institutional memory, 134
Insurance
  breaks in coverage, 46
  premiums for, 22
  transparency in, 67
  under- and uninsurance, 42–43, 45–46
Insurers, administrative costs and, 27
Intervention treatment, 90
Iron Triangle analogy, 17–18, 22

Japan, 12, 18, 19, 21. *See also* Toyota Production System (TPS)
Jones, Daniel T., 106
Joy, Bill, 134–135

Kellermann, A. L., 26
Kendal Corporation, 5–6
Kessler, Ronald, 115
Kirch, Darrell, 65–66

"Lean" principles, 12–13, 15, 105–109, 130
Levy, Paul, 63
Life expectancy (LE), 19, 20f

Magnetic resonance imaging (MRI), 28–29
Managerialism, models of, 69–70
Managing for Stakeholders (Freeman), 69
Marketing, to consumers, 28–29
Massachusetts General Hospital, 61
Massachusetts Health Care Quality and Cost Council, 65
Maternal mortality rate, 19
Mayo Clinic, 64
Media, news, 41, 48–49, 69–70, 83, 90–91, 101, 103
"Medical arms race," 28
Medical bankruptcy, 43–44
Medical device companies, 28, 63
"Medical home" concept, 117
Medical information sources, 48–49
Medical records, sharing of, 68
Medicare/Medicaid
  ambulatory surgeries and, 81
  cost inflators for, 22–24
  patient satisfaction with, 45
  pay-for-performance, 102
  spending, 63–64
  spending differentials, 77
Midwest Business Group on Health (MBGH), 114
Mission statements, 60–61
Mitchell, Ronald K., 84–85
Montefiore Medical Center, 64
Moral framework, for health care, 40
Moral hazards, 89, 126
MRI (magnetic resonance imagine), 28–29
Murman, Earll, 106, 108, 124

National Institute for Health and Clinical Excellent (NICE), 50
Nike, 136
Nonadherence, 47
Noorda, Ray, 3

Obesity, 24, 25f
Ohno, Taiichi, 76, 106, 130
Onboarding process, 15
Organisation for Economic Co-operation and Development (OECD), 19

Ostrom, Elinor, 139
Overuse, health care services, 29, 71, 75

Paperless environment, 118
Patient education, 28, 48–49
Patients, as stakeholder group, 13, 14
Patient satisfaction, 45
Payers, 13, 23, 81. *See also* reimbursements
Pay-for-performance, 102–103
Payment negotiations. *See* reimbursements
Peer group comparisons, 18
Personalized medicine, 30
Pharmaceutical companies, 4, 31
Physicians/doctors
  administrative costs for, 27
  on imaging utilization, 98f
  notes of, 68
  reimbursement of, 94–95
  satisfaction of, 48
  stakeholder alignment and, 4, 75
Pitney Bowes, 114–115
Population, aging of, 22
Porter, Michael, 8, 9, 88, 128–129
Prescription abandonment, 45
Preventable death rate, 19
Preventative medicine, 49, 90
Price/rate controls, 79. *See also* costs
Primary care specialists, shortage of, 26
Private health insurance, cost of, 22
Profit, stockholder, 11
Prostate cancer, 50
Providers, as stakeholder group, 13, 14
Purchasers, as stakeholder group, 13

Quality measures, 82

Radiology benefit managers (RBMs), 98f
Read, Leonard, 11
Reimbursements
  market presence, role of, 83
  to Medicare/Medicaid, 23, 65–66
  negotiations for, 78–80
  payers, fights with, 81
  performance link to, 102
  of physicians, 94–95
  on quality measures, 82
  treatment decisions and, 74
Return on investment, 11

"Safety net" system, 24, 44–45
Safyre, Steven M., 64
Saliency modeling, 62–66, 84–86, 104
Satisfaction, of patients/physicians, 45, 48, 89–90, 108
Screening tests, 99
Silos, concept of, 66–69
Single-payer systems, 50
Smith, Adam, 11
Societal expectations. *See* expectations about health
Stakeholder alignment
  creation of value and, 52–53
  enablers of, 131–133
  of goals, 4–6
  on payment negotiations, 74, 78–80, 133–134
Stakeholder conflict, 71
Stakeholder groups
  anthropological identification of, 59f
  coordination between, 14
  definitions of, 57–62
  Dependency Structure Matrix (DSM), 93
  "four Ps," 13
  managing for, 69–71
  mapping of, 104f
  onboarding process, 15
  ownership of health care crisis, 51
  qualitative classes of, 85f
  silo concept and, 66–69
  standoffs among, 31–32
  terms for, 60
  triggers for change among, 127
Stakeholder saliency, 62–66, 84–86, 104
Stakeholder theory, 8–9, 10–12, 127–131
Starbucks, 3, 4
Stuart, Toby E., 67
Suppliers, stakeholder alignment and, 4
Sustainability, long-term, 11

Tailored care, 29, 30
Tamoxifen, 29–30, 41
Tavistock group, 40

Teaching hospitals, 62–66
Technology, 28–31, 101–102
Teisberg, Elisabeth Omsted, 8, 9, 88
Towers Watson, 116–117
Toyota Production System (TPS), 12–13, 106, 130, 131
"Tragedy of the Commons" (Hardin), 8, 9, 108, 139
Trust, among stakeholders, 31–32, 78
Tufts Medical Center, 31–32

Underinsured, 42–43, 46
United Airlines, 3, 4
United Kingdom, 18, 19, 21, 40, 45, 47, 50
Uslan, Jody, 41

Value, in U.S. health care, 17–22
Value-based benefits design, 90
Value-chain model, 128–129
Value creation
  model for, 124f
  stakeholder alignment and, 52–53, 103, 105
  for stakeholders, 11
  through waste elimination, 76–78
Value proposition, 108. *See also* Cisco Systems
Vendors, stakeholder alignment and, 4
Viagra effect, 40–41
Voluntarism, philosophy of, 105
Von Hippel, Eric, 135–136, 138

Waste, in health care system, 76–78
Wellness programs, 116
Wikipedia, 57
Womack, James P., 106
Wood, Donna J., 84–85
Woolhandler, Steffie, 27
World Health Organization (WHO) rankings, 18

Zane, Ellen, 32
Zero-sum competition, 8–9